Yoga
for the
Joy of It!

Minda Goodman Kraines, MA

Professor, Mission College
Santa Clara, CA

Barbara Rose Sherman, BS

Registered Yoga Teacher (E-RYT 500)

JONES AND BARTLETT PUBLISHERS
Sudbury, Massachusetts
BOSTON   TORONTO   LONDON   SINGAPORE

World Headquarters

Jones and Bartlett Publishers
40 Tall Pine Drive
Sudbury, MA 01776
978-443-5000
info@jbpub.com
www.jbpub.com

Jones and Bartlett Publishers
Canada
6339 Ormindale Way
Mississauga, Ontario L5V 1J2
Canada

Jones and Bartlett Publishers
International
Barb House, Barb Mews
London W6 7PA
United Kingdom

Jones and Bartlett's books and products are available through most bookstores and online booksellers. To contact Jones and Bartlett Publishers directly, call 800-832-0034, fax 978-443-8000, or visit our website www.jbpub.com.

Substantial discounts on bulk quantities of Jones and Bartlett's publications are available to corporations, professional associations, and other qualified organizations. For details and specific discount information, contact the special sales department at Jones and Bartlett via the above contact information or send an email to specialsales@jbpub.com.

Production Credits
Acquisitions Editor: Shoshanna Goldberg
Associate Editor: Amy L. Flagg
Production Manager: Julie Champagne Bolduc
Production Assistant: Jessica Steele Newfell
Marketing Manager: Jessica Faucher
V.P., Manufacturing and Inventory Control: Therese Connell
Composition: Publishers' Design and Production Services, Inc.
Cover Design: Kate Ternullo
Assistant Photo Researcher: Meghan Hayes
Cover Image: © Alfred Wekelo/ShutterStock, Inc.
Printing and Binding: Malloy, Inc.
Cover Printing: Malloy, Inc.

Library of Congress Cataloging-in-Publication Data
Kraines, Minda Goodman.
  Yoga for the joy of it! / Minda Goodman Kraines, Barbara Rose Sherman.
      p. cm.
  Includes bibliographical references and index.
  ISBN 978-0-7637-6594-1 (pbk. : alk. paper)
  1. Hatha yoga. I. Sherman, Barbara Rose. II. Title.
  RA781.7.K684 2010
  613.7'046—dc22

                                                     2008054198
6048

Printed in the United States of America
13 12 11 10 09   10 9 8 7 6 5 4 3 2

To my husband, **Guy**,
and my children, **Marissa**, **Denaya**, and **Jesse**.
With love,
M. G. K.

To my husband, **Stu**,
my children, **Amber**, **Noah**, and **Abby**,
my beloved **mother** and **father**,
and my greatest yoga teacher, **Paramahansa Yogananda**.
With love and devotion,
B. R. S.

To our friendship,
which blossomed through
the writing of this book.
M. G. K. & B. R. S.

Brief Contents

Contents

Foreword

As a physician and psychiatrist I have pursued many different avenues of healing, yet yoga remains the most useful, time-tested, adaptable, and elegant system I have ever come across. It places the responsibility and the means for healing in the hands of the individual, where it belongs.

By good fortune, I came to the study of yoga 37 years ago. At the age of 18, I traveled to India to study with the great Indian yoga teacher T. K. V. Desikachar, and I have maintained a relationship with him ever since. His approach—passed down from his father, T. Krishnamacharya—individualizes the practice of yoga to fit the needs of each individual. The physical condition, emotional development, stage of life, and presence of illness guides the direction of the practice, allowing for modifications as changes occur. In this way, the practice becomes a kind and gentle approach to deepen self-knowledge as well as to maintain a body that is supple, youthful, and free from tension.

This lucid and practical text, *Yoga for the Joy of It!*, offers an introduction to one of the world's most ancient and reliable self-healing disciplines: the art of yoga. The Sanskrit root of the word yoga (*yuj*) means to yoke or connect, and through yoga we can truly connect with that which is best and truest in ourselves.

In this text, Minda Goodman Kraines and Barbara Rose Sherman—both longstanding practitioners and teachers of yoga—provide an enthusiastic yet evidence-based primer on the benefits, the spirit, the attitude, and the technical aspects of introducing yoga into one's life. Their language is simple and free from jargon. The reader can feel the delight they take in sharing their life-long passion for yoga, a discovery that, once made, often leads to a desire to make it available to others. The great teacher Krishnamacharya said it would be Western women who would carry yoga forward; in this text, we see his prophecy fulfilled.

— Reuben Weininger, MD

Preface

Imagine waking up in the morning feeling enlivened, happy, relaxed, and excited to begin your day. Imagine having clarity and composure during school exams. Imagine having satisfying relationships and fewer conflicts with your parents and loved ones. Yoga brings this into your life! A yoga class can make you sweat, relax, reflect, build strength, develop flexibility, and release emotions. This explains the widespread popularity of yoga today and the reason for this book, *Yoga for the Joy of It!*

In the 1960s and 1970s, yoga was mainly practiced by people with alternative lifestyles or people who were a part of the "young and hip" generation. Today, yoga is for everyone and everybody—young and old, slim and obese, liberal and conservative, pregnant women, and even people with systemic diseases. There are many styles and approaches to yoga; it is easy to find one that fits your individual needs.

Yoga, a scientific system of body movement, builds strength and flexibility throughout the body and provides needed stress release in this fast-paced world. Yoga is not only a workout, but also a "work-in," a way of living that is not separate from daily life. Scientific research at many universities across the United States reveals the health benefits and the mind–body–spirit connection inherent in yoga. "Sweat and pump" was the way to get fit during the 1980s and 1990s. Now individuals realize the holistic benefits achieved from yoga—a fit body, an awakened mind, and an enlivened spirit.

Yoga transforms the mind and body and affects how we approach life. Practitioners of yoga enjoy this conscious approach to living, breathing, moving, and thinking. This explains why yoga classes now are popular at colleges, community centers, senior centers, and YMCAs. Yoga studios have sprouted up throughout the world. Yoga is appreciated not only because it is good for the body, but because it also feels great during the actual practice. Positive results are immediate.

Yoga for the Joy of It! is geared towards the college-level yoga class and provides valuable information to enhance the yoga experience. It is the result of years of teaching thousands of students, practicing under the guidance of incredible teachers, and assimilating the yoga philosophy into our daily lifestyles. We have included every aspect of the yoga practice, from what to bring to the first class to the appropriate breathing techniques, how to meditate, and a brief history of this ancient tradition and science. The poses, called asanas, are described in full detail with their benefits, the correct alignment, and appropriate modifications. A thorough discussion of the correct posture needed for each yoga pose is presented as well as proper back care. The photos show proper form and balance. The appendices give options for pregnant, overweight, and older adults as well as guidelines for proper nutrition and healthy eating; helpful yoga resources and yoga books also are included. Finally, we designed worksheets to record medical history, evaluate posture and flexibility, and record daily yoga practice and nutritional habits.

This book makes yoga come alive. Student testimonials as well as inspirational quotes are sprinkled throughout the text. Boxes entitled "Yoga Science," which provide scientific research on yoga, are included in many of the chapters. The study questions and yoga moments at the end of each chapter help students understand the material and how they can utilize the information for their personal growth.

It is our hope that *Yoga for the Joy of It!* launches your exploration and joyful journey of yoga!

Acknowledgments

We deeply appreciate our first editor, Jacqueline Geraci, who launched our project of writing this book, and our new editor, Shoshanna Goldberg, who continued with the process. Special thanks to the fabulous team at Jones and Bartlett Publishers, including Amy Flagg, associate editor, Jess Newfell, production assistant, and Jessica Faucher, marketing manager.

We thank our yoga masters, Ganga White, Erich Shiffmann, Shiva Rea, John Friend, Seane Corn, and Tracey Rich, who profoundly contribute to the modern world of yoga.

We offer a big thank you and *namaste* to Richard McLaughin, Iyengar yoga teacher extraordinaire, for his insightful and precise teachings.

With gratitude, we recognize the efforts, enthusiasm, and expertise of George Welik, our photographer, and his lovely wife and assistant, Peggy.

We thank Mission College for the use of their facilities for our Northern California studio photo shoot. We thank Lais da Silva, owner, and Denise Zaverdas, assistant director, of the Santa Barbara Yoga Center for use of the sacred and beautiful studio space for our Southern California photo shoots.

We thank our wonderful yoga models in Northern California: Jesse Dailey, Denaya Kraines, Yi-Yu Lan, Cheong Leung, Korak Mitra, Jeffrey Samson, Tatiana Thomas, Thuy Truong, and Brenna Wundrum.

We thank our wonderful yoga models in Southern California: Maureen Clair, Anne Chenoweth, Damien de Bastier, Jason Edwards, Mario Gonzales, Karen Jacobs, Stu Sherman, Kim Stevenson, and Denise Woods.

We celebrate all of the marvelous yoga teachers who directly inspire and uplift us, and we thank all of our past, present, and future yoga students who continually enrich us on our path.

In gratitude, we honor our dear families and friends for their unconditional love and patience, and we send a virtual hug to our incredible husbands—Guy Kraines and Stu Sherman—for their hours of providing ideas, editing, and support.

Namaste,

Minda and Barbara Rose

About the Authors

■ Minda Goodman Kraines, MA
Professor, Mission College
Santa Clara, CA

Minda has been a full-time instructor at Mission College for 30 years. In addition to yoga, she has taught ballet, modern dance, jazz dance, choreography, aerobics, cardio-kickboxing, weight training, and body alignment and stretching techniques for personal trainers. She created a Fitness Professional Certification program at Mission College that is highly regarded and attended. She is the author of two other college texts that are both in their fifth edition, *Jump into Jazz: A Primer for the Beginning Jazz Dance Student and Beyond* and *Keep Moving: Fitness through Aerobics and Step.*

Minda has been studying yoga for 35 years and has taught yoga for 15 years. Her greatest yoga inspirations include Ganga White, Shiva Rea, Seane Corn, and Baron Baptiste. Although Minda has been teaching body movement for almost four decades, she continues to find new inspirations and keeps growing and learning as both a student and teacher. She holds a Bachelor of Science degree in theater from Northwestern University and a Master of Arts degree in dance from Mills College.

■ Barbara Rose Sherman, BS
Registered Yoga Teacher (E-RYT 500)

Barbara has practiced yoga and meditation for 30 years and has been teaching for 15 years. She has facilitated more than 25 yoga retreats in California and two yoga/meditation/hiking retreats in Italy. She also has generated websites, written educational films, and designed and presented corporate wellness programs. An article about her use of relaxation techniques in dentistry has been published in *Yoga Journal.*

Barbara's foundation of yoga is grounded in the teachings of Paramahansa Yogananda. A devoted practitioner, she has trained with Erich Shiffmann, Ganga White, and Tracey Rich. She also is certified in Therapeutic Yoga. Barbara teaches from her heart, illuminating the *spirit* of yoga.

She has served as a volunteer for Children's Hospital in Los Angeles and Direct Relief International. Committed to personal growth, Barbara continually takes courses in nutrition, neuroscience, and stress reduction. She integrates her love of science and yoga into her popular workshops, *How to Meditate, Pray, Heal, Peace and Prosperity in Challenging Times,* and *Women's Health and Healing.*

Barbara received her Bachelor of Science degree from the University of Southern California.

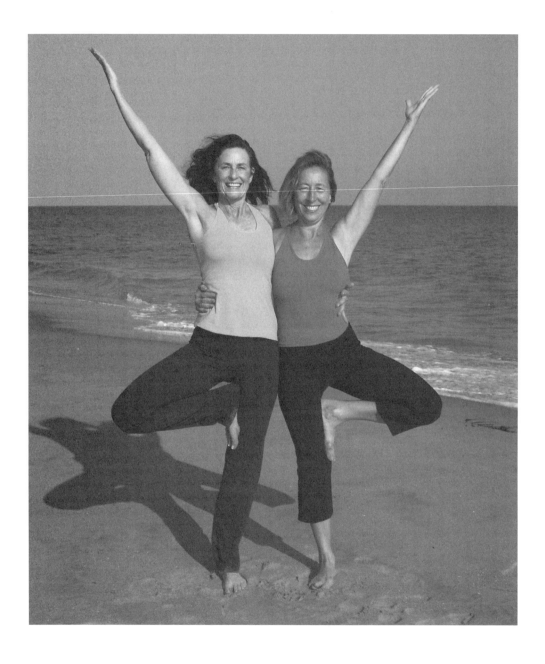

CHAPTER ONE

Start Your Yoga Journey!

Wake Up and Smell the Yoga!

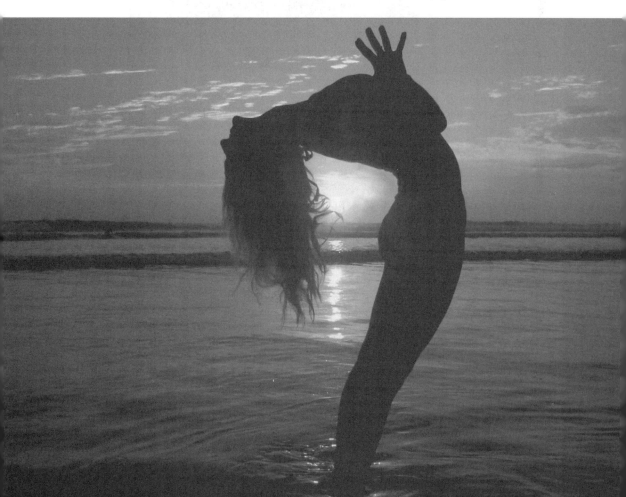

*Practicing asanas began to teach me about myself.
The body is such a great school of learning. It makes
me pay attention.*

— **Lilias Folan**

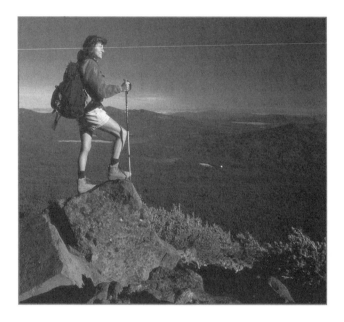

If this is your first yoga course, you are probably very excited but perhaps unclear about what to expect. This chapter helps to orient you to your first experiences on the value of yoga, appropriate attitudes to take in class, materials you will need for class, what to wear, and ways to have a successful practice.

WHY YOGA?

People come to yoga for many different reasons:

* To achieve flexibility
* To build strength
* To improve balance

- To heal an injury
- To reduce stress
- To relax

At the start of your yoga practice, it may appear that you are just putting your body through unusual positions. As you continue though, your body becomes more comfortable, and you feel subtle changes not only in your body but also in your approach to daily life. By consistently toning and stretching your body and relaxing your mind, you actually begin to feel more joy and calm on a regular basis.

Student Testimonial

"Since I began to practice yoga, I am stronger. I deal with life's difficulties more easily."

Just like any physical exercise, yoga challenges your level of fitness by improving your strength, endurance, and flexibility.

Yoga Science

The American Council on Exercise studied 34 women during an 8-week period. These women who practiced yoga three times a week for 50 minutes demonstrated the following improvements (Boehde & Porcari, 2005):

- Total body flexibility improved by 13% with significant results in trunk and shoulder flexibility.
- Muscular fitness improved by enabling group to do 16 more push-ups and 14 more curl-ups.
- Yoga participants experienced a 17-second increase in their one-legged stand time.

However, yoga goes beyond the sweat and muscle work of a typical fitness workout. It also integrates your mind, your body, and your unique essence or spirit.

> The heart of the yoga practice: Develops body awareness, improves fitness, and establishes a positive mental attitude.

As a student of yoga, you discover correct body alignment as well as how to maintain that alignment with minimal stress on your muscles and joints. Because yoga moves the body through all its possible positions, it has been scientifically proven to have a positive effect on all the systems of our body. By using your body in ways that your daily life does not demand, you dramatically influence all these systems that will in turn establish balance, health, and healing.

Yoga Science

According to the National Center for Complementary and Alternative Medicine of the National Institutes of Health, relaxation techniques, such as those practiced in yoga, can (Lipson, 1999–2000):

- Lessen chronic pain, such as lower back pain
- Lessen arthritis, headaches, and carpal tunnel syndrome
- Lower blood pressure and heart and breathing rates
- Reduce insomnia

Students of yoga also generally report:

- Higher levels of energy
- Decreased levels of stress and anxiety
- Increased feelings of general well-being

Yoga also encourages an accepting attitude of your strengths and limitations, without judgment or negativity. The time you spend practicing yoga can bring a new awareness not only to your body but to how you approach your life. This makes yoga not only a *workout, but also a "work-in"*!

THE YOGA ATTITUDE

The attitude you bring to your yoga practice dramatically affects your yoga experience.

Beginning yoga is an adventure that takes you on an incredible journey—the journey inward toward self-discovery.

"As a man thinketh in his heart, so he is." This quote by Solomon in *Proverbs* 23:7 reveals that the mind may be likened to a garden, which may be intelligently cultivated or be allowed to run wild. This corresponds to modern medical research, which proves that every thought, emotion, and action has a physiological response in your body.

Because our body's health and energy are affected by how we think, outlined below are some appropriate attitudes to experience and explore on your yoga journey. These attitudes weave together and create a wonderful mental tapestry for a successful yoga practice.

Gentleness

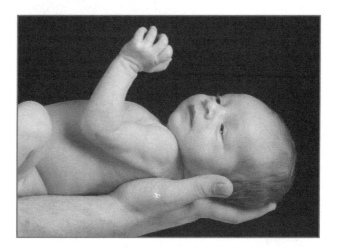

Your instructor will guide you through poses and techniques, but you are the true teacher. Only you know how these shapes and positions feel inside your body. Approach the class and poses with self-love and self-appreciation. What a joy to be able to move your body!

Each student in your class has different genetics, a different physical structure, and a different accident history, so with this in mind make no judgments about yourself as you approach your practice. Remember, the person standing next to you may have been a college-trained gymnast or may be someone who has suffered a back injury.

Always listen to your body's wisdom. Develop the ability to listen to the teacher within you. Honor your individuality!

 Tend to your vital heart, and all you worry about will be solved.

— **Rumi**

Openness

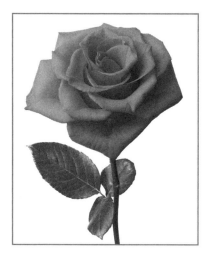

Be open to experiencing new feelings and to discovering moving your body in different ways.

 Yoga reaches parts of the body that we usually do not reach during a normal working day.

 Student Testimonial

"I sit at a computer for 8 hours a day. My body craves my yoga class, because I can stretch and nurture my back."

When the body is worked and massaged from the inside out, stagnation or "dis-ease" is eliminated. This allows circulation, nerve supply, and "ease" to be restored. Look at the two diagrams of rope (**Figure 1-1A** and **Figure 1-1B**). Let's imagine that the rope represents how a nerve impulse travels through the body.

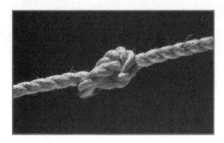

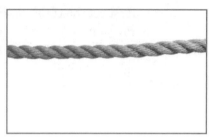

Figure 1-1A   **Figure 1-1B**

In the first rope the energy is knotted, so the impulse has difficulty traveling from one end to the other. The second rope shows how the nerve impulse can travel easily from one end to the other. Yoga practice opens the body and removes these "knots," facilitating free-flowing energy and health.

Respect

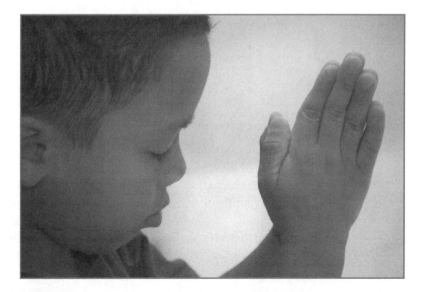

Keep your focus on your mat. Keep your eyes from wandering around the room so that you can center and concentrate inward on this moving meditation.

Respect the time class begins and plan to stay for the entire practice. If you come late, you will miss the beginning meditation. If you leave early, you will miss the final pose, Corpse pose, where the body integrates all the movements in a deep relaxation.

Respect your limitations. Never allow your body to move into pain.

Focus and Concentration

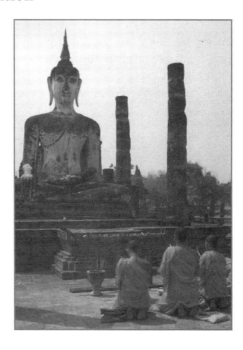

Weave together your focus and concentration each time you practice yoga. Enjoy and go inside, as you *in-joy* the wonder of moving with focus. We are in a culture where we multi-task, so enjoy the opportunity the yoga class provides to center the mind.

> **!** Yoga allows the body and mind to return to a normal and healthy pace by bringing awareness to the moment with concentration only on the breath and the posture.

Patience

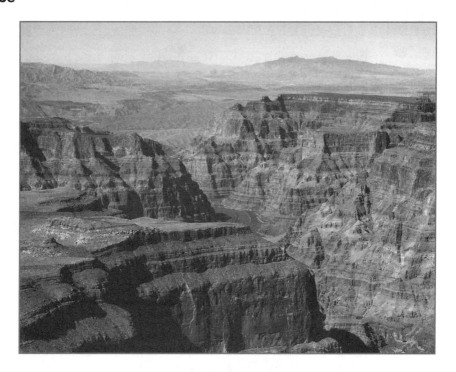

Think about the Grand Canyon. This wonder of the world was created by water, slowly! Be serene, self-accepting, and patient with yourself and your practice. Watch for subtle and dramatic changes in your daily life.

> **!** Mentally decide to give your best to every class, and with time your will see your body become stronger and more flexible.

> **Student Testimonial**
>
> *"Yoga gives me the chance to appreciate myself. I love the opportunity to be fully self-absorbed, giving my body the time and care it needs."*

MEDICAL CONSIDERATIONS

Before embarking on your yoga journey, consider a medical evaluation of your current health status. If you have been following a regular exercise program, a yoga class poses no problem. However, certain risk factors make it appropriate for the student to consult a physician and receive a medical clearance before beginning the yoga course. The following factors should be considered:

- Your age and level of activity. Men and women over 45 years of age who have never been involved in a regular exercise program may benefit from a checkup.
- Pregnancy. Women who are pregnant or who have given birth within the previous 3 months should be cleared by their doctor.
- A history of heart disease. The severity of the condition determines the appropriate level of exercise participation.
- **Hypertension**. This should not deter a person from participating in yoga, but a doctor's clearance is essential.
- **Arthritis**, diabetes, fibromyalgia, and cancer. This should not deter a person from participation, but a doctor's clearance is appropriate.
- Eye problems, like **glaucoma**, need to be cleared by a doctor because of the extra pressure to the eyes with inversions.

People with these conditions can certainly participate in a yoga program, but they are encouraged to visit a physician for medical clearance and to determine what precautions should be taken.

Once you are committed to begin, complete Worksheet 1: Medical Profile and return it to your instructor before you start the class.

A medical profile provides the instructor with the knowledge about your present health condition and other appropriate information to make your practice safe.

CLOTHING AND EQUIPMENT
Clothing

Comfortable clothing that allows ease of movement is essential when practicing yoga.

- Clothing should be nonrestrictive and preferably made of cotton. Cotton allows the body to breathe.
- Zippers and snaps on clothing should be avoided.
- Clothing should be fairly tight fitting so that the instructor can observe your form easily and make corrections when necessary. However, modesty should be observed.

Most women wear either dance pants or shorts or pants made specifically for yoga. The top can also be a standard workout top or a basic tank t-shirt. Men usually wear sweat pants, bike shorts, specific running shorts, or pants for yoga. The top is a basic t-shirt or tank t-shirt.

Support undergarments are extremely important when practicing yoga:

- Women should wear a sports bra that fits snugly and provides adequate support.
- Men may desire to wear athletic supporters for adequate support.

Most of this attire can be purchased at a sporting goods store or a clothing store specifically for yoga and dance. Your instructor may provide guidance on the yoga attire, but if the outfit provides freedom to move, it is usually appropriate.

- Jewelry is discouraged during the yoga practice because it can hinder ease of movement.
- Hair should be secured in a manner that does not distract or disrupt the student. Try to use hair accessories that will not get in the way when poses are performed on the back.
- Cell phones and pagers should be turned off during the yoga session.

- Food is also not appropriate in the yoga studio.
- Water is acceptable, but make sure the top is secured.

Props

In many yoga classes, props are used to ease the poses and create more success. These props may be available in your studio, but if they are not available, you may want to purchase them:

- Sticky mat (**Figure 1-2**)
- Blankets (**Figure 1-3**)

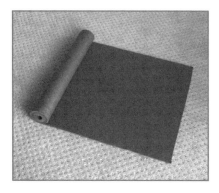

Figure 1-2

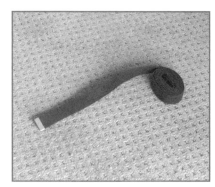

Figure 1-3

- Blocks (**Figure 1-4**)
- Strap (**Figure 1-5**)

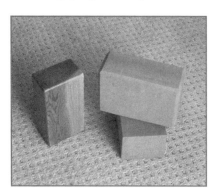

Figure 1-4

Figure 1-5

- Bolsters (**Figure 1-6**)
- Eye pillows (**Figure 1-7**)

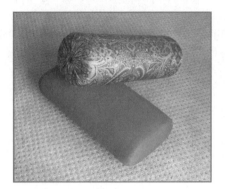

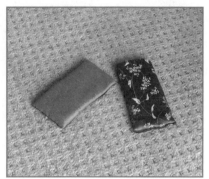

Figure 1-6   **Figure 1-7**

STRUCTURE OF A YOGA CLASS

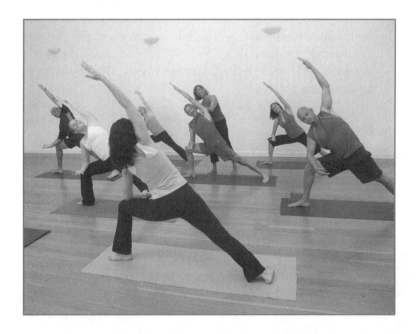

Opening Awareness

Your instructor usually begins by having you sit on a mat, perhaps with a blanket to elevate your hips for comfort. Then you are given cues to achieve correct alignment. This is followed by a few minutes of breathing or mediation practice that allows you to arrive in the room, in the moment, and in your body. This time facilitates clearing the distractions of the day and opens you to what follows next.

Opening Stretches

These stretches warm and bring circulation into various muscles and joints, gradually preparing your body for the more strenuous aspect of the practice. Most often these are done sitting, on all fours, or on your back. Frequently, this is the time in class when core strength movements are performed.

Standing Poses

Many classes begin the standing sequence with Sun Salutations, a flowing series of postures that create heat, stability, and strength in the body. Once the body is warm, and perhaps a slight sweat has occurred, traditional standing poses are executed. Standing poses build leg and core strength while teaching correct body alignment and principles of balance and poise.

Balance Poses

Once the body is warm and the mind is fully focused on the practice, balance poses become the next challenge. Breath, strength, and flexibility are all integrated in these balance poses, which require willpower, concentration, and discipline.

Floor Poses

On the floor, back bends and forward bends are executed. All these poses are aimed at creating a healthy back because these poses twist, compress, and stretch the spinal column. This brings circulation to the spinal muscles and stimulates the nerve supply that ultimately brings radiant health to the body!!

Inversions

This is when you turn your body upside down. In these poses, gravity is reversed and your organs, bones, and muscles are rejuvenated. In addition, **endorphins**, the "happy hormones," are secreted that create a sense of well-being in the mind and body.

Relaxation

This is the yoga dessert! Your body now assimilates all the movements you have practiced during the class and is able to deeply rest. The deep relaxation that occurs during this segment of your practice profoundly affects your nervous system and helps to eliminate stress and extraneous thoughts.

CHECKLIST FOR A SUCCESSFUL YOGA CLASS

- It is best to practice yoga on an empty stomach. Try not to eat at least two hours before class because the body functions more efficiently if it is not busy digesting food. On a full stomach, the oxygenated blood flows toward the digestive system instead of the joints and muscles.
- Be on time. In fact, arrive ten to fifteen minutes early to prepare your body and mind for the practice ahead. Yoga classes are structured with a beginning, a progression of poses, and a relaxation time. Please allow for the full class time.
- Dress comfortably for maximum movement as well as relaxation. This causes the blood flow, breath, and movement to be easy and unrestricted.
- Clear your mind of outside interference when you enter the classroom. Be prepared to fully concentrate on the lesson.
- Find a place to put your mat where you can easily see and hear the instructor. Allow yourself plenty of space so you can stretch freely.
- Be sensitive to any of your injuries. Pay attention to the injured area during your early arrival time as well as during the practice.
- REMEMBER, YOUR BODY IS DIFFERENT FROM EVERYONE ELSE'S BODY. DO NOT COMPARE YOURSELF WITH ANYONE ELSE IN THE CLASS.

- *Listen to your body.* Every day your body has a different amount of energy. Honor this uniqueness. If you cannot do some poses, work on them slowly, gradually, and patiently. Always come out of a pose when your breath or equilibrium is disturbed or there is strain in your body.
- Movement and breath are coordinated together. This integration of breath and movement is essential to yoga. Take deep, diaphragmatic breaths, inhaling and exhaling through the nose.
- Most importantly, stay in the moment during your yoga practice. This ability to stay in the moment will flow into your daily life, creating clarity, balance, and joy for yourself and others you come in contact with each day!

Whatever you can do, or dream you can do, begin it. Boldness has genius, power and magic in it. Begin it now.

— Goethe

THE YOGA ALPHABET

We have designed a yoga alphabet as a fun and insightful tool for understanding the breadth and depth of yoga. This introduces you to the ways and means yoga will enrich your life and why you will be happy you have made the initial commitment to practicing yoga.

A = alignment	N = nurturing
B = breath	O = openness
C = concentration	P = posture
D = discipline	Q = quiet
E = energy	R = relaxation
F = focus	S = strengthening
G = grace	T = tension-free
H = holistic	U = unify
I = introspective	V = vitality
J = joyful	W = wonderment
K = kinesthetic awareness	X = x-citing
L = lightness	Y = yogi
M = mindfulness	Z = zest

The alphabet is an additional way to find meaning in your yoga practice. Each of the words will come alive as you go deeper into your yoga practice and experience what you can learn from the consistent awareness of your body and breath. One way to use this alphabet is to focus on one of the words during your practice and then to bring its meaning into your daily life.

This attention to concepts will enrich your yoga practice!

STUDY QUESTIONS

1. What are your expectations from this yoga class?
2. Why is yoga a "work-in" as well as a workout?
3. According to the National Institutes of Health, what are three health benefits of yoga?
4. What three attitudes can you bring to your yoga practice?
5. Who needs a medical exam before embarking on yoga?
6. Outline a typical yoga class.

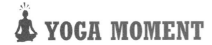

YOGA MOMENT

Create your own yoga alphabet and observe your feelings as you create this alphabet.

CHAPTER TWO

Breathing for the Joy of It!

Breathe in Health and Happiness

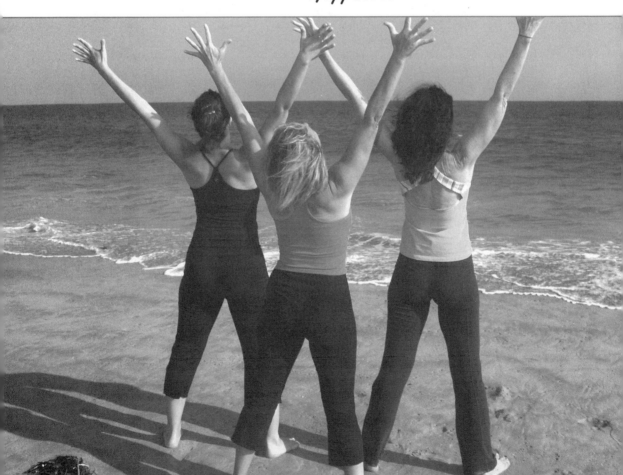

When the breath wanders the mind also is unsteady. But when the breath is calmed the mind too will be still, and the yogi achieves long life. Therefore, one should learn to control the breath.

— **Svatmarama,** *Hatha Yoga Pradipika* **(ancient text on yoga)**

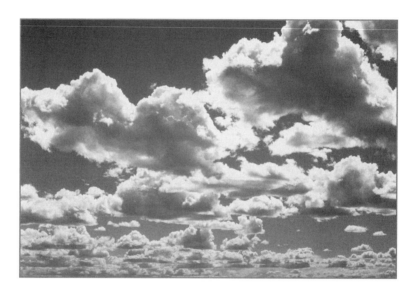

THE MIRACLE OF BREATH

Breath is life. We can survive weeks without food, days without water, but only moments without breath. When a baby is born the breath establishes life, and at the final moments of death the breath leaves the body. The breath bridges the external world and the internal world. In this chapter you learn how to take full advantage of this simple yet profound life-supporting act. The word *spiritus*, in Latin, and the word *ruach*, in Hebrew, both mean breath and life energy (Weil, 1995, pp. 203). When you bring in breath, you bring in life force.

The average person takes in a minimal amount of oxygen when breathing. The result of this type of breathing is tightness throughout the body, stress, and a lowered immune system. Other than musicians, athletes, and singers, few people are aware that the abdomen should expand during inhalation to supply the cells with adequate amounts of oxygen. Learning slow yoga breathing dramatically affects the nervous system and the quality of life.

PHYSIOLOGICAL BENEFITS OF PROPER BREATHING

- Improves stamina
- Improves digestion
- Improves circulation
- Strengthens the immune system
- Oxygenates the tissues
- Enhances concentration and focus
- Decreases anxiety
- Promotes a sense of well-being in body and mind

Proper breathing is a master key of health and positively affects the entire body (Krucoff, 2000).

Student Testimonial

"Practicing yoga breathing has made me calmer and more energetic. I do not get out of breath when I am rushing to class!"

THE YOGA BREATH

For thousands of years, yogis have recognized the power of the breath. They developed techniques to harness this power. Techniques of breath control are called **pranayama**. This word is a combination of two Sanskrit words, *prana*, meaning life force or breath, and *yama*, meaning control. To attain peace and enlightenment, yogis practiced many breathing techniques. Before describing the specific yoga breathing, it is beneficial to first observe your natural breathing cycle.

To gain awareness of your natural breath cycle, perform the following exercise:

- Lie down on your back with your knees bent and the soles of the feet fully rooted on the floor.
- Observe your natural breathing process.

- Do you take in a lot of air?
- Does the breath fill only your chest or does it flow into your abdomen?
- Does the air gush out all at once?
- Do you fully empty your lungs before taking in the next breath?
- Do you feel tension in the shoulders when you breathe?
- Do feel any constriction in your body when you breathe?
- Make mental notes of these observations.

THE DIAPHRAGMATIC BREATH

Once you have completed the observation of your natural breath cycle, it is time to learn diaphragmatic breathing, an important element in the practice of yoga.

- Find a comfortable seated position.
- Place your hands on the diaphragm with the fingertips facing each other and the middle fingers touching.
- Breathe in through the nose in a slow, steady stream.
- Visualize the air flowing into the lungs, inflating the diaphragm like a balloon.
- Feel your hands moving outward (**Figure 2–1A**).

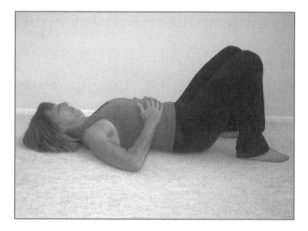

Figure 2-1A

- Slowly exhale through the nose in a steady stream.
- The diaphragm will deflate like a balloon and the hands will move inward (**Figure 2-1B**).

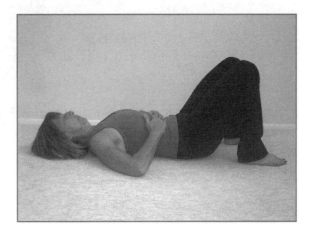

Figure 2-1B

- For the next inhalation, place the hands on the side ribs. Initially the diaphragm will inflate; then observe the movement of the ribs outward.
- On the exhalation, feel the side ribs moving inward.
- For the third inhalation, place the fingertips on the collarbone (clavicle). Observe the diaphragm inflate, and then the side ribs expand. Finally feel the subtle movement of breath under the fingertips.
- On the exhalation, feel the collarbone release.
- Practice the three-part diaphragmatic breathing on the floor, on a chair, against a wall, in the car, walking to class, walking your dog, everywhere!!

Smile, breathe, and go slowly.

— Thich Nhat Hanh, Vietnamese monk nominated for the Nobel Peace Prize

Qualities of the Breath

Fast Breathing	Slow Breathing

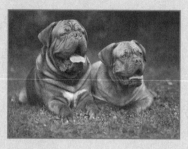 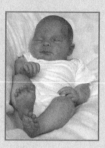

Fast Breathing	Slow Breathing
Shallow	Deep and regular
Excites	Calms
Louder	Quieter
Produces anxiety	Produces relaxation

Yoga Science

Andrew Weil, director of the Program of Integrative Medicine and professor of clinical medicine at the University of Arizona in Tucson, teaches breath work to all his patients and states the following:

"I have seen breath control alone achieve remarkable results: Lowering blood pressure, ending heart arrhythmias, improving the long-standing patterns of poor digestion, and increasing blood circulation throughout the body, decreasing anxiety and allowing people to get off addictive anti-anxiety drugs and improving sleep and energy cycles" (Krucoff, 2000).

UJJAYI BREATHING

The word **ujjayi**, in Sanskrit, means *victorious*. This type of breathing anchors the yoga practice. In fact, just practicing this breath without practicing the asanas brings vibrancy and vitality to the body. The ujjayi breath combines the deep-flowing diaphragmatic breath with a sound that is created in the back of the throat. This sound, like a whisper, similar to the sound of the ocean or Darth Vader's voice in *Star Wars*, vibrates in the back of the throat. The sound of the ujjayi breath, like music, affects the ears, jaw, mouth, and eyes.

Similar to the diaphragmatic breath, the ujjayi breath also consists of three parts. When inhaling through the nose, the breath first fills the diaphragm, then the rib cage, and then the upper portion of the chest. The inhale and exhale are equal in length, which relaxes the nervous system. Additionally, the ujjayi breath brings strength to the diaphragm and the core muscles while increasing the internal temperature of the body. Yoga practitioners consciously use the ujjayi breath to build strength, discover balance, and establish a rhythmic flow to the asana practice.

When utilizing the ujjayi breath throughout the entire practice, especially in the transitions between asanas, the whole yoga session becomes a moving meditation.

Follow the sequence below to experience the ujjayi breath.

- Find a comfortable seated position.
- With your mouth open, take breath in through your mouth and make a "ha" sound as you inhale and exhale.
- Now, close your mouth and create the same "ha" sound in the back of the throat, as you inhale and exhale through your nose.
- Make the inhale slow, smooth, and steady.
- Create an exhale that mirrors your inhale, slow, smooth, and steady. This balanced rhythm of the breath soothes the nervous system while calming and relaxing the mind.

Breathing in I calm the body and mind

Breathing out I smile

Dwelling in the present moment

I know this is the only moment

— Thich Nhat Hahn

ALTERNATE NOSTRIL BREATHING

This *pranayama* breathing technique in Sanskrit, called *nadi shodhana*, cleanses and balances the energy channels of the whole body (**Figure 2-2**). It also dramatically soothes the nervous system while stimulating both hemispheres of the brain. In this process, both nostrils clear, the blood receives more oxygen, and the mind becomes calm and lucid. Follow the sequence described to experience alternate nostril breathing.

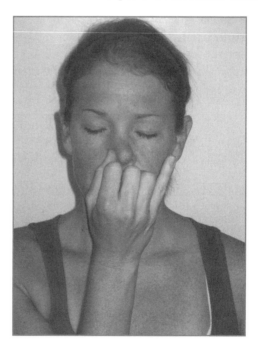

Figure 2-2

- Sit comfortably on the floor or on a chair extending the spine and opening the chest.
- Take the index, middle, and ring fingertips of the right hand toward the palm (**Figure 2-3**).
- Gently close off the right nostril with the thumb.
- Inhale slowly and smoothly through the left nostril.
- Pause.
- Close off the left nostril with the baby finger while removing the thumb from the right nostril and exhale slowly and smoothly.

- Inhale through the right nostril.
- Pause.
- Remove the fingers from the left nostril as you exhale.
- Repeat this sequence by inhaling through the left nostril.

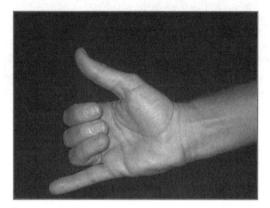

Figure 2-3

Several variations of hand positions and breathing rhythms slightly alter the effects of this process, and all variations work! When practicing this *pranayama* technique, visualize a life force plus the breath flowing into your body and brain.

VISUALIZATIONS FOR PRACTICING THE YOGA BREATH

Yoga combines breath awareness and movement. Each breath during a yoga practice possesses the ability to transform. Keeping the focus on the breath enriches the yoga experience! The breath is the most important aspect of the practice.

Experiment with these visualizations:

- Visualize the diaphragm as a balloon. As you inhale, the balloon inflates. As you exhale, the balloon deflates.
- Inhale health, light, and joy. Exhale toxins, tension, and resistance.
- Inhale length and openness. Exhale tightness and constriction.
- As you breathe in, notice areas of tension. As you breathe out, release the tension.
- Use the inhale to observe. Use the exhale to accept.

- Use the inhale to lift and expand the pose. Use the exhale to go deeper into the pose.
- Think of the breath as a circle. Connect the inhale and exhale seamlessly.
- In yoga practice make the inhale and exhale mirror each other in length, texture, and quality.

If the breathing becomes labored or short, lessen the intensity of the pose and reestablish a smooth and steady breath. Remember, like the asanas, yoga breathing takes practice. Observe, explore, and experience joy!

STUDY QUESTIONS

1. List four benefits achieved with proper breathing.
2. Define:
   a. *Pranayama*
   b. Ujjayi
   c. *Nodi shodhana*
3. Record your observations after watching your natural breath cycle for three minutes.
4. Describe two visualizations to use with the yoga breath.
5. What makes the ujjayi breath unique?

YOGA MOMENT

Observe yourself tense, nervous, or upset in a situation. Consciously turn your attention to slow diaphragmatic breathing. Record your observations.

CHAPTER THREE

Meditation for the Joy of It!

Enter Into Quietude

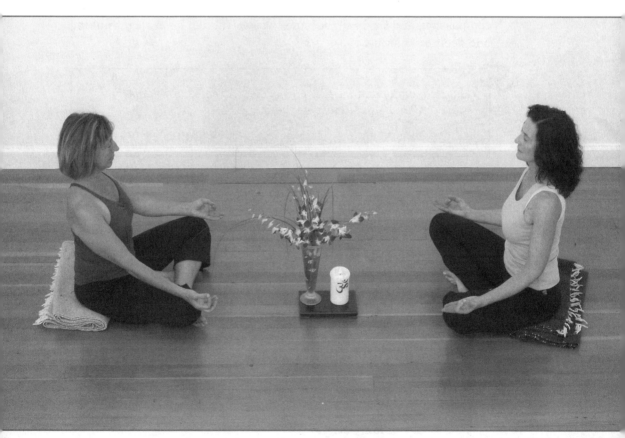

Even a little bit of this practice will save one from dire fear and colossal suffering.

— *Upanishads* (ancient Hindu text)

DISCOVER YOUR TRUE NATURE

Yoga asanas target the spine, making it strong so that the student can sit still during meditation. The mind, like a wild horse, runs wildly, thinking between 25,000 to 50,000 thoughts in a day (Marano, 2001). Scientists say that many of those thoughts are negative and are repeated from the previous day. Also proven is the connection between thoughts and reality—what we think is what we attract into our lives. Controlling a restless mind brings clarity, calm, and creativity into life. When the mind is quiet, we learn to live our lives with greater wakefulness and compassion, and the brain becomes a powerful tool for critical thinking and decision making.

The state of the mind is a vicious cycle. It creates problems for itself, and then tries to resolve them.

— Swami Phajmarpad

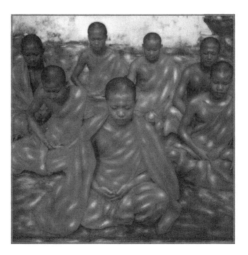

Figure 3-1

"For more than 2,500 years, Buddhist monks have known that practicing meditation leads to increased strength, calmness and self-awareness, strengthened contact with sub-consciousness feelings and thoughts and greater spiritual growth" (Edwards, 2006) (**Figure 3-1**). A team of Harvard medical scientists, led by Sara Lazar, PhD, a researcher at Massachusetts General Hospital, found that meditation could also alter the structure of the brain. The study revealed an increased thickness of the regions of the brain associated with attention and processing sensory input (Cullen, 2006).

Time Magazine devoted an issue to the science and practice of meditation. "Scientists study it. Doctors recommend it. Millions of people—many of whom don't even own crystals—practice it every day. Why? Because meditation works" (Stein, 2003). Several articles present various medical studies that reveal meditation increases immune system function, improves cardiovascular health, and reduces hypertension (high blood pressure).

Erich Schiffmann, in his book *The Spirit and Practice of Moving into Stillness* (2006, pp. 4, 305–327), says, "The practice of yoga is the practice of meditation—or inner listening. . . . It's a matter of listening inwardly for guidance all the time, and then daring enough and trusting enough to do as you are prompted to do. . . ."

Yoga Science

Herbert Benson, a graduate of Harvard School of Medicine and a pioneer in mind–body medicine, studied many individuals for months and discovered the benefits of meditation that he defined as the **relaxation response**. The main physiological features of the relaxation response are:

- Lower blood pressure
- Lower heart rate
- Lower levels of lactic acid
- More alpha waves (this frequency of brain waves is associated with relaxation)

Dr. Benson states, "The relaxation response is a physical state of deep rest that changes the physical and emotional responses to stress . . ." (Benson, 1975, pp. 1–79). Meditation heals!

Meditation removes the sludge and film over the mind and uncovers our true nature, which is joy, peace, and bliss. When you clean a dirty windshield with glass cleaner and a paper towel, it takes more than one wipe to achieve sparkling clear glass. The process often makes the windows seem dirtier. Mediation is like a cosmic glass cleaner. It works scientifically and marvelously to eventually clean and clear the window of your mind.

MEDITATION BASICS

In the Bhagavad-Gita the spine is referred to as a well-strung bow. The string represents the spine and the curved wood represents an open heart. The alignment of the spine is essential to the meditation posture. **Figure 3-2**, **Figure 3-3**, and **Figure 3-4** show examples of good meditation postures.

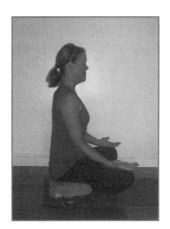   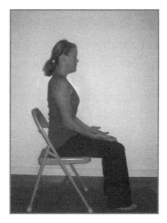   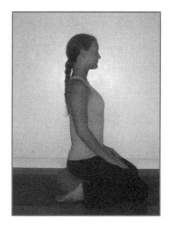

Figure 3-2   **Figure 3-3**   **Figure 3-4**

MEDITATION POSTURE

- Sit in a comfortable position on the floor or on a chair.
- Close the eyes.
- Align the back of the sacrum with the back of the head.
- Stack the vertebrae one on top of the other, creating space and awareness.

- Lengthen through the crown of the head.
- Open the chest by moving the underneath portion of the armpits forward.
- Draw the shoulder blades down the back.
- Let the hands rest comfortably on the thighs with palms up or down.
- Relax the eyes away from the lids and release the brows.
- Soften the skin on your face.
- Relax the entire body yet keep the spine straight and vibrant.
- Allow the focus to go inward.

By meditation we connect the little joy of the soul to the vast joy of the spirit.

— **Paramahansa Yogananada, *Spiritual Diary*, Self Realization Fellowship, Los Angeles, CA**

MEDITATION TECHNIQUES

The art of meditation is both observing wandering thoughts and having the control and ability to bring the attention back to the moment. Meditation practice trains the mind to be present. The four meditation techniques described below provide the structure for this experience. Explore each technique and find the ones that work best for you.

Following the Breath Meditation

- Sit in the meditation posture.
- Relax your body.
- Set an intention to follow your breath—so simple yet so profound.
- Begin to concentrate on the breath as in comes in and out through the nose.
- Watch the breath, without controlling it.
- Observe its natural rhythm.
- Allow the breath to deepen without forcing it.

- If thoughts appear or the attention wanders into the future or the past or to sensations, gently bring your awareness back to the breath.
- Initially, practice this meditation for five minutes.

Mantra Meditation

A **mantra**, a sound repeated over and over again, may be used as the focus in meditation. The sound becomes one with the consciousness. The most common sound used in this type of meditation is **OM**, the universal mantra. This **Sanskrit** term translates as *oneness*. Other Sanskrit mantras that can be repeated are *So Ham*, which honors the light and the dark; *Sat Nam*, which means truth; and *Shanti, Shanti*, which means peace, peace. Non-Sanskrit words such as mother, grace, or love may also be repeated in this meditation.

- Begin in the meditation posture with the eyes closed.
- Relax the body, and then begin to repeat the chosen sound or mantra.
- If the mind wanders, bring the awareness back to the mantra.
- Initially, practice this meditation for five minutes.

Expanding Love Meditation

- Begin with correct meditation posture.
- Relax the body and relax the mind with several minutes of slow circuitous breathing.
- Feel the goodness and compassion of your heart. Be grateful for this. Feel self-love and self-acceptance.
- Expand these feelings to your immediate family.
- Expand these feelings to all people in the community.
- Expand this love and acceptance to people all over the world.
- Feel your love and kindness spreading like a sphere of goodness in all directions.
- Spend at least five minutes in this meditation.

Visualization Meditation

- Begin in the correct mediation posture.
- With the eyes closed and the body alert yet relaxed, bring to mind a physical place of pleasure and healing, such as a special beach,

a mountain top, a rushing river, a quiet meadow, or a beautiful garden.

- Visualize every aspect of this place: the smell of the ocean, the color of the sky, the sound of the birds, the feel of the wind on the body, the taste of the salt air, and the overall sensation of restfulness and peace that this location brings.
- Allow these sensations to embrace and calm the mind and body.
- Like any meditation, distractions will occur. Return to this peaceful vision.
- Spend at least five minutes in this meditation.

WHERE AND WHEN TO MEDITATE

Many yoga classes begin and end with a short period of meditation (**Figure 3-5**). Continue your practice at home by creating a sacred space in

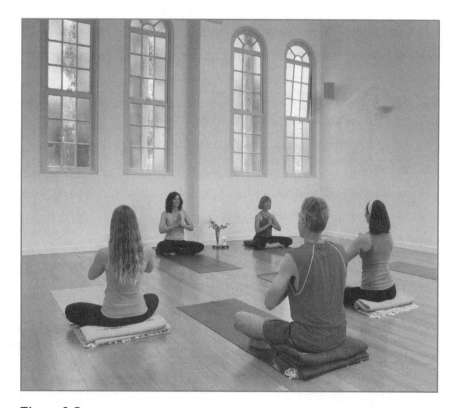

Figure 3-5

your home that is quiet and pleasing. It can be part of a closet, an area of the bedroom, a room specific for yoga and meditation, or an outdoor sanctuary. Returning to the same place creates positive vibrations and trains the mind and body for the experience ahead. Many meditators enjoy making an altar with photos of spiritual teachers and loved ones, quotes, flowers, or other meaningful objects.

- Intend to meditate at the same time every day.
- Be consistent with the chosen time.
- Start with five minutes.
- As the practice strengthens, gradually increase meditation time until twenty minutes is achieved.

Anyone who practices can obtain success in yoga but not one who is lazy. Constant practice alone is the secret of success.

— Hatha Yoga Pradipika

Problems When Meditating

Practitioners of meditation usually experience the same basic problems during meditation:

Problem	Solution
The body moves and itches	Keep meditating
Distractions take the stage	Keep meditating
Insecurity—Am I doing this properly?	Keep meditating
Difficult to retain a focus	Keep meditating

If any of these problems arise during the practice, and undoubtedly they will, maintain an accepting attitude. Let go of tensions and tightness. Relax and bring awareness back to the breath, the mantra, or the visualization. Consistent practice reaps amazing benefits.

When the life of a man, freed from all distractions, finds its unity in the spirit, the knowledge of the infinite comes to him immediately and naturally, like a light from a flame.

— **Rabindranath Tagore**

BENEFITS OF MEDITATION

- Improved focus
- Greater joy
- Openness of heart
- Greater presence in the moment
- Inner vibrancy
- Greater compassion
- Less internal conflict
- Less stress
- Greater attunement with nature
- *You add to this list!*

Create calm during meditation and watch it filter into every aspect of life: health, relationships, job, creativity, and more!!

Little by little, through patience and repeated effort, the mind will become stilled in the Self.

— **Bhagavad-Gita**

PRACTICAL WAYS TO UTILIZE THE BASIC MEDITATION IN A BUSY LIFE

- Before you leave for school, to positively visualize the day
- Before an exam, to establish mental clarity and concentration

- Before an athletic event, to gain calm and focus
- Before a presentation, to create dynamic energy
- During work, instead of coffee, to recharge the body's battery
- Before attacking a problem, to discover creative solutions
- During an emotional conflict, to gain perspective and control
- When agitated, aggravated, and anxious, to create calm
- When feeling unconfident, to empower
- Before sleep, to ensure a restful evening and to reflect on the day with gratitude
- Every day for more "in-joyment" of life!

STUDY QUESTIONS

1. State four physiological changes in the relaxation response.
2. Describe your favorite meditation technique.
3. What are two problems encountered during meditation and how can you handle them?
4. Describe in detail the meditation posture.
5. How can meditation be a tool in your life?

YOGA MOMENT

Find a quiet place in nature where you will be undisturbed. Sit in a meditation posture. Relax and close your eyes. Begin to listen to the sounds around you. Be like an antenna—receptive—allowing sounds to enter your awareness . . . traffic, birds, talking. Hone in on these sounds. Listen attentively. Then transfer this listening to the sound of the breath. Stay with listening to the breath for five minutes. Note any sensations or feelings of quietness or calm. Open your eyes and record your observations.

CHAPTER FOUR

Yoga Alignment

Be Grounded

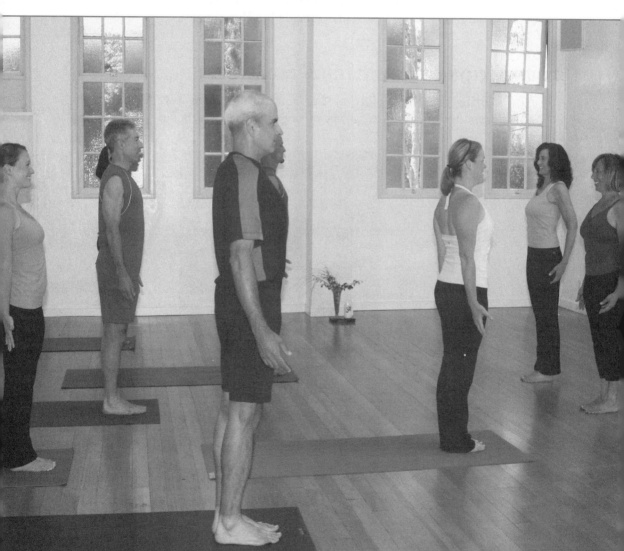

Mountain pose teaches us, literally, how to stand on our own two feet . . . teaching us to root ourselves into the earth. Our bodies become a connection between heaven and earth.

— **Carol Krucoff, RYT (registered yoga teacher)**

This chapter focuses on correct body alignment by thoroughly examining every aspect of Mountain pose—Tadasana. You will understand how energy flows through every yoga pose and how an awareness of this energy flow strengthens your yoga practice. A discussion of postural deviations and proper back care is also included in this chapter.

FOUNDATION OF ALIGNMENT: TADASANA

Bring to mind a picture of a mountain (**Figure 4-1**). Visualize the mountain's grandeur, power, strength, steadiness, beauty, and balance.

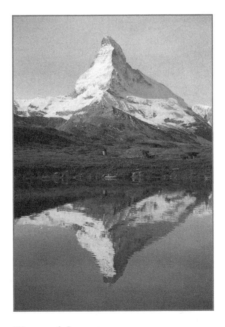

Figure 4-1

These qualities create the essence of Tadasana. With the continual practice of Tadasana, your body becomes strong and properly aligned and your mind becomes steady. The structure of Tadasana is inherent in all standing yoga postures, and elements of Tadasana are found in all yoga poses. Therefore, a thorough understanding of this posture is essential. To understand Tadasana, let us build this pose from the bottom up.

- *Root the feet*
  - Classically, this pose is performed with the feet together, big toes touching. If you have back issues, tight hamstrings, or find this position uncomfortable, then keep the feet hip distance apart.
  - Root evenly through the four corners of each foot.
  - Distribute the weight evenly between the inner and outer edges of both feet and lift the arches.
  - Make sure the feet point directly forward, with the toes spread wide, and stretch and lengthen each toe on the mat.
- *Lengthen the legs*
  - Keep the ankles balanced directly over the heels, not allowing them to roll in or out.
  - Fully straighten the legs by lifting the kneecaps upward. You can feel this action by placing your fingertips on the fleshy part above your kneecaps and lifting the skin upward. This movement engages the quadriceps (muscles on the front of the thighs) without locking the knees. The knees can slightly bend if your hamstrings are tight or your back is tender.
  - Roll the knees outward so that the center of the kneecap lines up with the second toe.
  - Roll the thighs inward to activate the inner thighs. You can experience this engagement of the inner thighs by placing a rolled blanket or a yoga block between the thighs and squeezing.
- *Position the pelvis*
  - In Tadasana, the pelvis, which is the cornerstone of alignment, must be in a neutral position. Here are cues to help you understand what "neutral" means.
    - Imagine the hipbones as headlights on a car—shine them directly forward.

- Your pelvis is like a bucket of water, filled to the very top. If you tilt it forward or backward, the water will spill. Maintain the position where the water is stable.
- Keep the pelvis level by drawing an imaginary straight line from one hip bone to the other.

- *Activate the abdominals*
  - Draw the abdominal muscles inward and upward.
  - Imagine pressing the navel toward the spinal column.
- *Close the ribcage*
  - Draw the ribcage inward toward the spine and lift the sternum.
  - Imagine you are wearing a very tight vest with buttons. If you extend outward with the ribcage, the buttons will burst!
- *Relax the shoulders*
  - Draw the lower edges of the shoulder blades together to open the chest.
  - Create as much distance between the ears and shoulders as possible.
  - Release all tension in the shoulders.
  - Hang the arms freely from the shoulders.
- *Lengthen the neck and lighten the head*
  - Balance the front and back muscles of the neck.
  - To achieve this balance, lengthen the back of the neck and slightly draw the chin toward the throat.
  - Keep the chin parallel to the ground and not jutting forward.
  - Let your head be light, like a helium balloon. Feel it lengthening away from the neck.
  - Softly gaze straight ahead.
  - Relax the facial skin without furrowing the brow or clenching the jaw.
- *Extend the arms*
  - Let the arms hang downward by the body, with the fingers pointing down.
  - Roll the upper arms outward with the elbows reaching toward the back of the room. This allows the chest to comfortably open.
  - Keep the arms close to the sides with space at the armpits.
  - The palms can either face forward or inward toward the thighs.
  - The fingers are together in a relaxed position.

Experiencing this correct alignment in Tadasana creates balance, grace, and lightness in the body and a sense of peace and harmony in the mind.

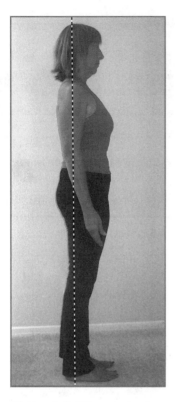 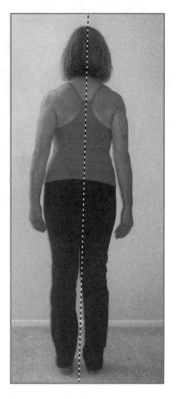

Figure 4-2 Alignment reference points from the side

Figure 4-3 Alignment reference points from the back

Here are the ideal reference points as viewed from the side for Tadasana (**Figure 4–2**):

- Center of the ear
- Center of the shoulder
- Center of the hip
- Behind the kneecap
- In front of the ankle

Here are reference points as viewed from the back for Tadasana (**Figure 4–3**):

- Middle of the head
- Center of all vertebrae
- Cleft of the buttocks
- In between the heels

Student Testimonial

"I often practice Tadasana when I am waiting in a store line. It keeps me centered and brings yoga into my daily life."

The alignment found in Tadasana not only exists in the structure of every standing pose, it also is inherent in almost all yoga poses (**Figure 4-4**)!

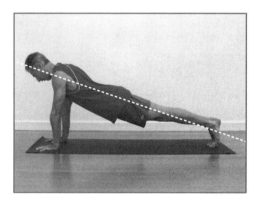

Figure 4-4 Observe the structure of Tadasana in Plank pose

LINES OF ENERGY

You are probably aware of *energy* as it flows throughout your body. As you are reading this paragraph, you may feel lively, sluggish, or somewhere in between. The amount of energy you put into each pose enhances your yoga practice. By focusing specifically on how energy moves through each pose, you achieve a more dynamic pose and heighten your body awareness.

To get a sense of how energy actually moves through the body, start by holding your arm out in front of you. Begin by sending a moderate current of energy out your arm. Now intensify this current. Now lessen the current. Pretend that the intensity of the current is on a dimmer switch and you have the control to increase or decrease the energy output.

Let's look at the foundational pose, Tadasana, and see how this concept of "**lines of energy**" can enhance your practice of this pose. First, no matter what pose we are referring to, all lines of energy radiate from the core and travel through the torso and the extremities. The diagram of Tadasana shows two arrows or two lines of energy. One goes from the navel toward the head, lifting the torso, neck, and head upward toward the sky and another arrow begins at the navel and goes downward rooting your hips, legs, and feet to the earth (**Figure 4-5**). Poses that extend the body in many directions have several lines of energy (**Figure 4-6**). Remember, all lines of energy start at the core.

Practice standing in Tadasana and experiment with sending just the right amount of current or energy in two directions.

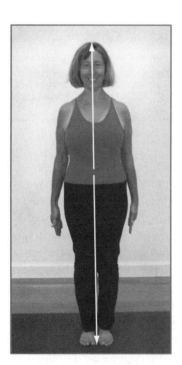

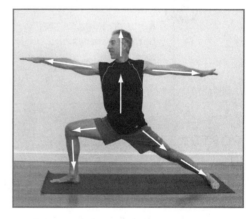

Figure 4-6 Observe multiple *lines of energy* in Warrior II

Figure 4-5 Two lines of energy in the Tadasana pose

Joel Kramer, in his classic article "Yoga as Self-Transformation" (1980), states five ways in which awareness of lines of energy improve your yoga practice:

1. Increase energy within the posture
2. Tone and relax the nervous system
3. Decrease the likelihood of injury caused by overextension of muscular stretch
4. Increase strength and endurance in postures
5. Internally align the body in the pose

In any pose, when you strengthen the energetic current along the lines, the body is able to align itself from the inside out. When the posture is properly aligned, you feel a sense of freedom and expansion in the shape. By bringing consciousness to these available energy currents, you align the joints properly, which in turn reduces risk of injury and encourages maximal muscular extension. You will come to appreciate this concept of energy lines as you continue to progress through your yoga practice.

> *Keeping your energy active makes the body radiant and vibrant in the postures and prolongs youthfulness. The awareness and posture you cultivate will carry over from yoga practice to daily life.*
>
> **— Ganga White**

POSTURAL DEVIATIONS

Tadasana is the body's posture perfectly aligned. When the body does not maintain the alignment as described in Tadasana, postural deviations occur. Because our alignment is habitual, most people are not aware when they are out of alignment. When a person has maintained a misaligned spine for his or her entire life and then tries to find correct placement, the position will feel odd and uncomfortable. It takes both muscular reconditioning and kinesthetic awareness of the correct alignment to change. By concentrating on the appropriate alignment cues as defined in this chapter, practicing Tadasana and regularly performing **asanas** that stretch and strengthen the appropriate muscles, an individual can improve his or her posture and alignment.

There are three primary postural deviations: lordosis, kyphosis, and scoliosis. All are concerned with the alignment of the spinal column. All three can be temporary or permanent. They may be caused by fatigue or by a muscle, tendon, or ligament imbalance, which stretching and strengthening can correct. If the deviations are caused by structural "abnormalities" of the bones, exercising will not improve the condition. In this situation, a physician should be consulted.

In Tadasana there are natural or "neutral" curves in the spinal column (**Figure 4-7**). These curves minimize the excess stress on the spinal column and its surrounding musculature. In a deviation, a curve becomes excessive.

Lordosis is an excessive curve of the lumbar spine (**Figure 4-8**). In this position the pelvis has an increased anterior tilt, which increases the normal inward curve of the lower back. This spinal deviation is often accompanied by a protruding abdomen and buttocks, rounded shoulders,

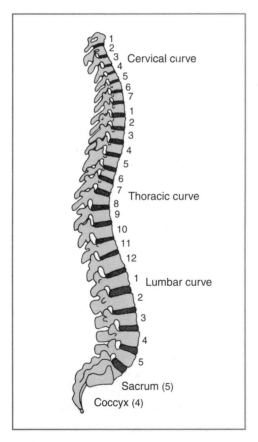

1
2
3 Cervical curve
4
5
6
7
1
2
3
4
5
6
7 Thoracic curve
8
9
10
11
12
1 Lumbar curve
2
3
4
5
Sacrum (5)
Coccyx (4)

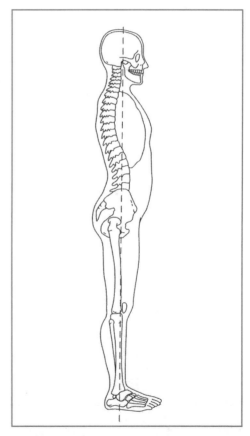

Figure 4-7 Natural curves of the spinal column

Figure 4-8 Lordosis
Source: Kraines, Minda Goodman & Esther Pryor. (2004). *Jump Into Jazz*, Fifth Edition. New York: McGraw Hill. Reprinted with permission.

and a forward head. Often, this deviation is caused by poor postural habits and can be corrected with body awareness and the practice of yoga asanas.

Kyphosis is an increase in the outward curve of the thoracic spine (**Figure 4-9**). It is usually accompanied by round shoulders, a sunken chest, and a forward head. Poor postural habits are usually the cause of this deviation. Sitting at a desk for many hours in a day can exaggerate this posture. Practicing yoga asanas can help to alleviate this condition.

Scoliosis is a lateral curve of the spine (**Figure 4-10**) and cannot be seen from the side like the other two deviations. Usually, the forward

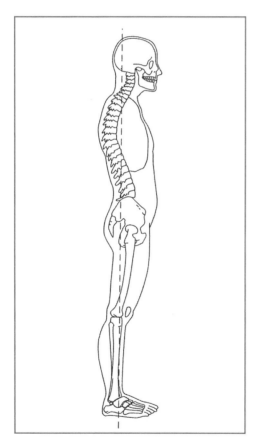

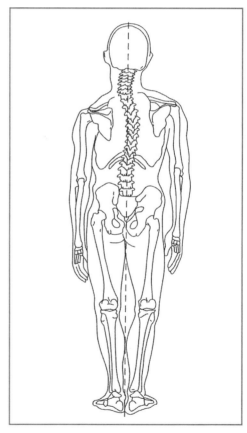

Figure 4-9 Kyphosis
Source: Kraines, Minda Goodman & Esther Pryor. (2004). *Jump Into Jazz*, Fifth Edition. New York: McGraw Hill. Reprinted with permission.

Figure 4-10 Scoliosis
Source: Kraines, Minda Goodman & Esther Pryor. (2004). *Jump Into Jazz*, Fifth Edition. New York: McGraw Hill. Reprinted with permission.

bend position in yoga can detect the imbalance of the spine, where one side of the spinal column is higher than the other side. Viewing the body from the front can reveal one hip or one shoulder higher than the other. If this issue is structural, a physician should be consulted. Often though, habits such as carrying a baby on the hip or a heavy purse over one shoulder can cause the deviation.

If you were to carefully analyze how you carry out daily activities such as sitting, standing, carrying objects, and sleeping, you would understand how poor postural habits develop. By performing activities with a minimum of strain on the muscles and joints, alignment can improve and lower back pain can be alleviated (Kraines & Pyror, 2004, pp. 45–47).

Student Testimonial

"I used to wake up every morning with a backache. My yoga practice has taught me so much about the care of my back that this is no longer an issue."

BACK CARE

Many people study yoga because of lower back pain. A healthy back is one of the goals of the yoga practice. The asanas move the spine in all positions to stretch and strengthen the muscles and joints. If you do experience back pain, this section of the chapter outlines causes and ways to manage and alleviate the pain (Schatz, 1992, pp. 1–20).

Causes of Lower Back Pain

Many factors can produce lower back pain. Prolonged sitting—an occupational hazard for many—can create unnecessary tension in the lower back by causing the vertebral muscles to shorten and become inflexible while encouraging weak abdominal muscles.

Poor postural habits are another culprit of lower back pain. When the muscles of the spine are continually held in imbalance, the lower back muscles excessively contract to hold the spine in a vertical position.

Faulty body mechanics can cause excess stress on the back. Lifting objects with the legs straight and holding objects far from the body are two mistakes that can injure the lower back.

Minimal physical activity exacerbates back pain. Weakened abdominal muscles, lower back tightness, and excess weight are all contributors. This situation causes the pelvis to tilt forward, resulting in undue pressure on the lower back (Vad, 2004, pp. 3–15).

> Yoga helps alleviate back pain by consciously aligning the body, strengthening the abdominal muscles, and creating flexibility in the spinal muscles.

Outlined below are specific yoga movements that can help relieve lower back pain.

Asanas to Improve Lower Back Flexibility

- Knee to Chest pose (Apanasana, Chapter 10)
- Supine Twist pose (Jathara Parivartanasana, Chapter 10)
- Child's pose (Balasana, Chapter 12)
- Seated Forward bend pose (Pascimottanasana, Chapter 9)
- Head to Knee pose (Janusirasana, Chapter 9)
- Cat/Dog pose (Chakravakasana, Chapter 9)
- Legs Up the Wall pose (Viparita Karani—without bolster variation, Chapter 12)

Hold each of these poses for five breaths. Legs up the wall may be held for up to five minutes.

Asanas to Improve Abdominal Strength

All four of these abdominal exercises strengthen the muscles in a slightly different manner. Perform all four!

■ Yoga Sit-Up (Figure 4-11)

- Lie on the back with the legs extended to the ceiling.
- Place a yoga blanket that has been folded to a small size in between the inner thighs.
- Squeeze the blanket.

- Place the hands behind the head with the elbows flat to the floor and the thumbs flat on the jaw.
- Inhale.
- As the shoulders and head lift off the floor, exhale.
- Do not let the elbows roll in—keep them in the same position that they were in on the floor.
- Keep the lower back firmly in contact with the floor.

Modify by performing with one leg extended and the other leg with the knee bent and the sole of the foot on the floor. Repeat ten times and rest. Eventually, build up to two sets of yoga sit-ups.

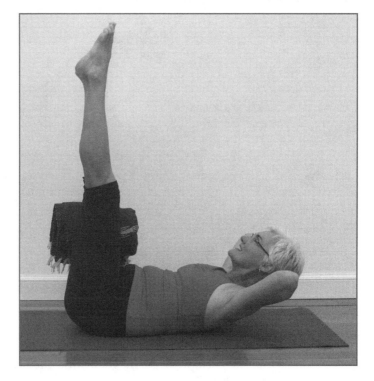

Figure 4-11 Yoga sit-up

■ Yoga Bicycle (Figure 4-12)

- Lie on the back with the knees at the chest and the hands behind the head with the elbows stretched outward on the floor.

- Inhale as you lift the head and shoulders off the ground.
- Exhale as you extend the left leg straight out without touching the floor. Simultaneously rotate the left elbow to the right knee.
- Keep the lower back fully in contact with the floor.
- Inhale when both knees are in toward the chest.
- Exhale as the elbow rotates to the opposite knee.

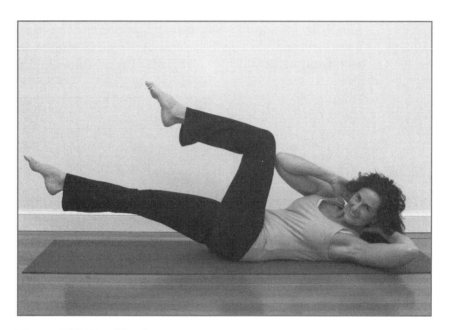

Figure 4-12 Yoga bicycle

■ Double Yoga Crunch (Figure 4-13)

- Start on the back, with the hands behind the head and the elbows flat on the floor.
- Inhale in this position.
- Exhale, as the knees lift toward the nose and the nose lifts toward the knees.
- Make sure the buttocks lift off the ground and the elbows stay open.

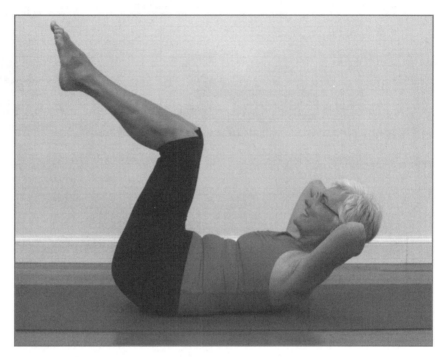

Figure 4-13 Yoga crunch

■ **30–60–90 Yoga Abdominal Strengthener (Figure 4-14)**

- Lie on the back with the palms under the buttocks facing the ground.
- Keep the neck long by drawing the chin close to the chest.
- Lift both legs 30 degrees from the floor and hold for ten seconds.
- Lift both legs 60 degrees from the floor and hold for ten seconds.
- Lift the legs 90 degrees and hold for ten seconds.
- Reverse and hold the legs at 90 degrees, 60 degrees, and 30 degrees.
- To modify, perform one leg at a time.

To alleviate lower back pain, perform these exercises daily. Even more important than the exercises is the awareness of correct alignment. Practice Tadasana regularly. Make it your habitual posture. Perform daily tasks with correct form. Use the knowledge you gain from your yoga practice to keep your body balanced and healthy!!

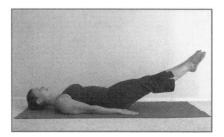 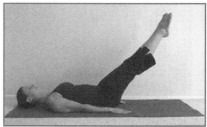

Figure 4-14A 30°   **Figure 4-14B** 60°

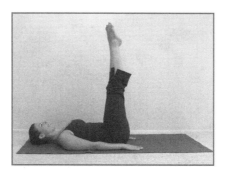

Figure 4-14C 90°

STUDY QUESTIONS

1. List four alignment cues for Tadasana.
2. State the reference points of Tadasana as viewed from the side.
3. Discuss three ways that *lines of energy* can enhance your yoga practice.
4. Look at the photo of Triangle pose (see Figure 6-2 in Chapter 6). How many lines of energy exist in this pose?
5. What are the three deviations of the spine?
6. What are three exercises that can help alleviate back pain?

 # YOGA MOMENT

Practice Tadasana in three different environments, such as the beach, the grocery store, and a park. Observe and record what you feel.

CHAPTER FIVE

Practicing the Postures

Welcome Challenges With a Breath and a Smile

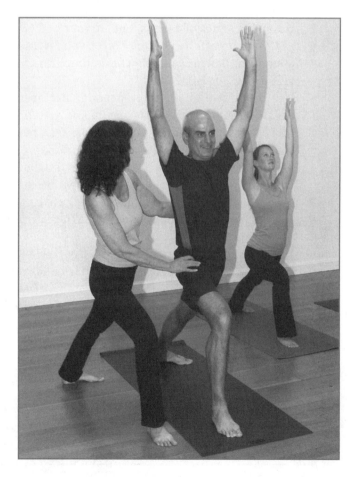

You should do the asanas with vigor and at the same time be relaxed and composed.

— **B. K. S. Iyengar**

Because yoga was developed in ancient Indian times, all terms used in the practice of Hatha Yoga are described in the ancient Indian language called Sanskrit. The Sanskrit word for a yoga posture or pose is "asana."

GUIDELINES FOR PRACTICING ASANAS

- Always listen to your body's wisdom. Your instructor will guide you through a series of asanas, but let your body be the teacher.
- Let your breath be the anchor of your asana practice. Establish a smooth, flowing, and rhythmic diaphragmatic breath. NEVER HOLD YOUR BREATH!!
- Use the inhale to lengthen, expand, and open the asana. Use the exhale to go deeper into the asana and soften the resistance.
- Move slowly into the poses, never forcing a position.
- Rest in Child's pose (see Figure 12-1 in Chapter 12) when the breath becomes labored or the body becomes fatigued.
- Initially, poses are held for just a few breaths. As your practice advances, the poses can be held longer (five to eight breaths).
- Be sensitive to your injuries and weaknesses, adapting any position to your body's needs.
- If your back or hamstrings are tight or tender, keep the knees soft.
- Learn the difference between discomfort and pain. NEVER ENTER THE PAIN ZONE!!
- Yoga is not a competition with anyone else or with yourself.

After each pose is described, suggestions for modifications are noted. Because every body is unique, it is important to discover the best variation of the pose for you!

> Experience joy and fulfillment in your yoga practice by focusing on the moment and not on success or failure.

USING THE PROPS

Although many props can be used in the yoga practice, we describe the most useful items that can facilitate ease in achieving the asana. These props are also readily available and reasonably priced. Additionally, you can find household substitutes for each. For health reasons obtain your own mat and props.

Yoga Blanket

Certainly, any blanket or beach towel would suffice, but blankets specifically for yoga are available at online sites or yoga schools (see Appendix C). Blankets that are appropriately folded can be used to elevate the hips in seated poses, to support the neck in lying poses, to cushion knees, and to pad or support any injured areas (**Figure 5-1**).

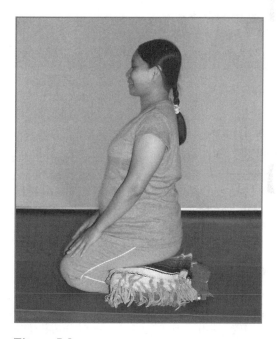

Figure 5-1

Yoga Block

This prop is available in wood or foam. The wood is firmer and the foam has more give, but the choice is personal. You can also use a phone book or dictionary. The blocks are primarily used in standing and seated poses to add extra length to the lower arm. The block is also used for support during lying poses (**Figure 5-2A** and **Figure 5-2B**).

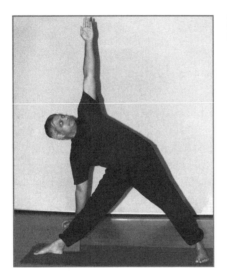

Figure 5-2A

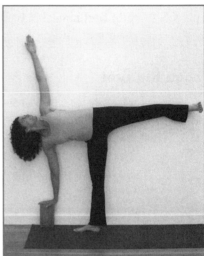

Figure 5-2B

Yoga Belt or Strap

The typical yoga belt is a heavy-duty cotton strap. You can certainly substitute a classic necktie or bathrobe belt. The belt is used as a way to increase your range of motion in forward folds, shoulder and leg stretches, and in any pose where you want to achieve greater flexibility than you can naturally attain (**Figure 5-3**).

Yoga Bolster

This prop can be found online or at a yoga store. It is used mostly in restorative poses to support the body. There are two styles, round or flat. We prefer the flat bolster because it is more comfortable for the back (**Figure 5-4**).

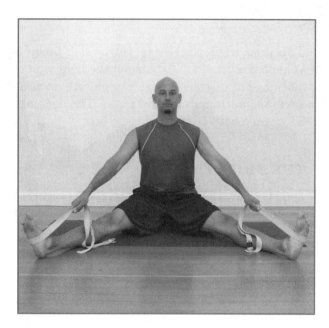

Figure 5-3

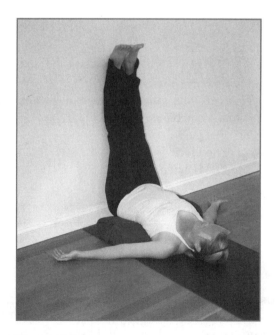

Figure 5-4

Eye Pillow

This prop, when placed over the eyes or brows, relaxes the nerves and enhances relaxation. It shuts out the light, quieting the optic nerve and blocking out distractions. It is wonderful to use during the final relaxation and during restorative poses. The contents of the eye pillow may be scented with lavender (Figure 5-4).

THE DRISHTI

During your asana practice the eyes are directed at a specific point to enhance concentration and attention. This point of focus is called the **drishti**. In Sanskrit drishti means "to see." By keeping the eyes gazing on one point, the mind eventually becomes steadfast and still. Each asana usually has a specific drishti, which is included in the asana descriptions. One drishti point mentioned is the **third eye**. The third eye refers to a point between the eyebrows, also known as the inner eye. Yogis believe bringing awareness to this point leads to expanded consciousness. Be mindful to your body and know that variations for the drishti are acceptable.

STUDY QUESTIONS

1. What are four guidelines to follow when practicing yoga asanas?
2. What is the benefit of using:
    a. The yoga strap?
    b. The block?
    c. The bolster?
    d. The eye pillow?
3. What does "drishti" mean?

 # YOGA MOMENT

Using a yoga strap, a necktie, or a piece of rope, hold it in front of your body and slowly raise it over your head. Your hands will slide outward to accommodate the stretch. Hold this stretched position for five breaths. Release the strap and record your observations.

CHAPTER SIX

Standing Poses

Be Strong

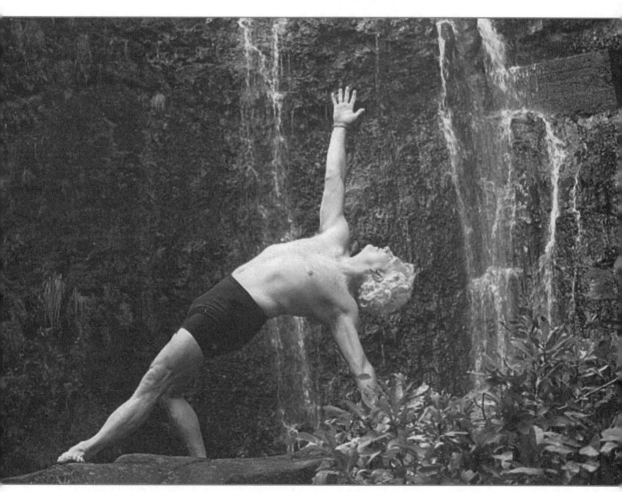

The basic difference between an ordinary man and a warrior is that a warrior takes everything as a challenge, while an ordinary man takes everything as a blessing or a curse.

— **Don Juan**

The principles of Tadasana are integral to the practice of every standing pose. Bringing strength, vitality, and balance to the body, the standing poses create and maintain a healthy spine. They also stretch and strengthen the muscles of the legs and encourage the core muscles to be fully activated. All the standing poses increase the body's need for oxygen. This creates additional stress on the heart and boosts blood circulation to often-neglected areas of the body, such as the joints, connective tissue, and internal organs. Oxygen is a source of nourishment to every cell; therefore an increased flow of oxygen to all parts of the body improves general health!

GENERAL ALIGNMENT TIPS FOR ALL STANDING POSES

- Keep toes long with the mound of all toes flat against the ground.
- Always track the knees in line with the second and third toes.
- Keep hips in neutral position and in line with each other.
- Engage abdominal muscles.
- Telescope the ribcage upward, keeping it pressed against the spine.
- Keep neck long to avoid any pressure on the cervical spine.

Student Testimonial

"I thought I was strong as a runner. Since practicing yoga and increasing my flexibility, I feel even more strength and power in my legs."

UTTANASANA: FORWARD FOLD POSE

Description

- Start in Tadasana, with feet touching or hip-width apart.
- Keep spine in neutral position.
- Hinge from the hip joints.
- Bend as far forward as you can, keeping spine and neck long (**Figure 6–1A**).
- Place hands on floor, toes, ankles, shins, knees, or thighs.
- From the straight back position fold over, bringing the forehead as close to the legs as possible (**Figure 6–1B**).

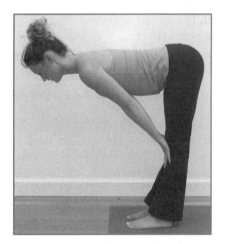

Figure 6-1A

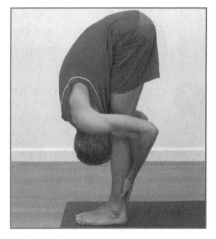

Figure 6-1B

Drishti

Initially, the gaze is at a point between the eyebrows (the third eye), which lengthens your spine. When you are in a full forward fold, the gaze is toward the knees.

Alignment Cues

- Feet touch or are hip-distance apart, depending on flexibility.
- Root through the four corners of the feet.

- Lift the kneecaps by engaging the quadriceps muscles.
- Roll the thighs inward.
- Stack hips, knees, and ankles in one vertical line.
- Spread the sit bones and lift them toward the ceiling.
- Kiss the forehead to the knees, releasing the neck and back muscles.

Benefits

This pose will:

- Lengthen and stretch the hamstrings and inner thighs
- Strengthen the legs and ankles
- Strengthen and stretch the spinal muscles
- Relieve upper body tension
- Calm the nervous system by placing the head lower than the heart

Modifications or Ways to Make the Pose Work for You!

- Keep knees soft if any back or hamstring issues.
- Hands hold elbows or interlace hands behind back for increased stretch.
- Perform against the wall for more support.
- Place a block by the toes if you cannot touch the floor.
- Place a block between the inner thighs to engage the inner thigh muscles.
- Place the top of your head on a block to release the neck muscles and support the head.
- Stand close to a wall and place the hands on it at waist height, then walk away from the wall until the torso is parallel to the floor.

UTTHITA TRIKONASANA: TRIANGLE POSE
Description

- Begin in Tadasana.
- Jump or step the feet 3 to 4 feet apart.
- Extend the arms parallel to the floor.
- Turn your right foot out a perfect 90 degrees.
- Turn your left foot in about 15 degrees.

- Reach fully to the side with the right arm.
- Bring the right arm to the shin, ankle, floor, or block.
- The left arm extends upward toward the ceiling, palm facing forward and in line with the right arm (**Figure 6-2**).
- Repeat asana on other side.

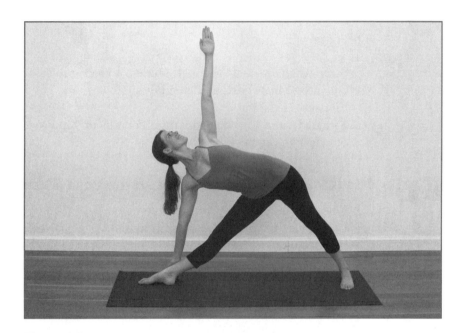

Figure 6-2

Drishti

The gaze is upward toward the extended arm, neutral (straight forward), or down at the floor. Listen to the feedback of your neck muscles.

Alignment Cues

- Root the feet firmly, emphasizing the connection of the outside of the back foot to the ground.
- Lift the kneecaps up to straighten legs and engage the quadriceps.
- Make sure that the heel of the front foot is in line with the arch of the back foot.
- Revolve the trunk forward and up.
- Create equal length on both sides of the ribcage.

- Imagine that your entire spine is flat against a wall.
- Send your tailbone toward the back heel.
- Align your hands with your shoulders.
- Create a straight line with your top and bottom arms.

Benefits

This pose will:

- Strengthen and tone the feet, ankles, knees, and legs
- Open the hips, chest, and shoulders
- Elongate the spine
- Stimulate and tone the abdominal organs and improve digestion
- Strengthen the neck

Modifications or Ways to Make the Pose Work for You!

- Keep knees soft if any back problems.
- Use a block behind the front shin to make the pose more accessible (**Figure 6–3**).

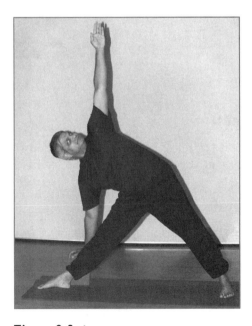

Figure 6-3

- Slowly extend the upper arm over the head for increased stretch.
- Practice using a wall to encourage proper spinal alignment.

VIRABHADRASANA I: WARRIOR I POSE

Description

- Start in Tadasana.
- Step the left foot back about 3 to 4 feet.
- The left toes turn slightly outward.
- The right foot stays facing forward, parallel to the sides of the mat.
- Keep both shoulders and hips facing forward.
- Revolve the left hip forward.
- Bend the right knee so the knee tracks over the ankle and is in line with the second and third toes.
- The back leg is straight with the back heel and baby toe flat against the floor.
- The arms extend over the head with the palms facing each other (**Figure 6-4**).
- Repeat the asana on the other side.

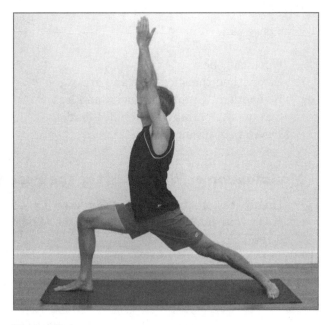

Figure 6-4

Drishti

The eyes look upward toward the hands, unless this is too strenuous for your neck. If so, look forward.

Alignment Cues

- Ground the back heel solidly into the mat.
- Press firmly into the big toe mound of your front foot.
- Lift the quadriceps.
- Move the tailbone downward.
- Tilt the pubic bone toward the navel.
- Bring the left hip bone forward and the right hip bone back.
- Telescope your ribcage upward.
- Evenly stretch the arms upward.
- Draw the shoulder blades down the back.
- Make sure the front knee tracks directly over the second and third toes.

Benefits

This pose will:

- Open the chest
- Strengthen the shoulders and arms
- Strengthen the ankles, knees, and legs
- Stretch the calves and Achilles tendon
- Develop endurance

Modification or Ways to Make the Pose Work for You!

- Create less of a bend in the front knee if you have knee problems.
- Keep your hands on your waist if the shoulders or neck are over-stretched.

- Place a blanket or block behind the back heel if the calf muscles are tight.
- Humble Warrior (**Figure 6-5**) can be performed to increase shoulder and chest flexibility.

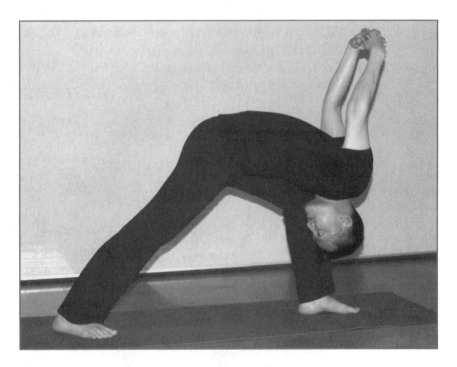

Figure 6-5

" > **Student Testimonial**

"Yoga makes me feel healthy, strong, and limber, which boosts my self-image and self-confidence."

VIRABHADRASANA II: WARRIOR II POSE

Description

- Start in Tadasana.
- Jump or step the feet approximately 4 to 4½ feet apart, with the arms extended to the sides and the palms facing the ground.
- Turn your right foot out a perfect 90 degrees.
- Turn your left foot in 15 degrees.
- The heel of the right foot is in line with the arch of the left foot.
- Bend your right knee, tracking it between the second and third toes.
- Turn your head to look over the right hand (**Figure 6-6**).
- Repeat the asana on the other side.

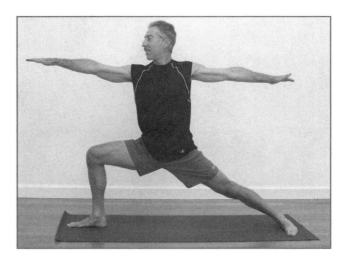

Figure 6-6

Drishti

The gaze is out over the middle finger of the front arm.

Alignment Cues

- Press the feet equally and firmly into the ground.
- Firmly root the baby toe side of the back foot.
- Align the shoulders directly above the hips.

- Work toward making the front thigh parallel to the floor.
- Let the tailbone heavily drop toward the floor.
- Draw the ribcage in as though you were wearing a tight vest.
- Move the chin slightly in toward the throat.

Benefits

This pose will:

- Strengthen the back and legs
- Intensely stretch the groin
- Open and strengthen the musculature of the hips
- Tone the abdominal muscles
- Build stamina

Modifications or Ways to Make the Pose Work for You!

- Take a narrower stance.
- Decrease the bend of the knee, but keep the knee tracking over the second and third toes.
- Practice with your hands on your hips.
- Reverse Warrior: Reach the back arm down toward the straight leg. Raise the forward arm. Gaze can be under the armpit or down toward the back leg (**Figure 6–7**).

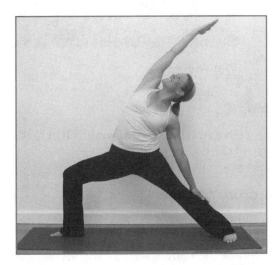

Figure 6-7

UTTHITA PARSVAKONASANA: SIDE ANGLE POSE

Description

- Stand in Tadasana.
- Jump or step your feet 4 to 4½ feet apart.
- Turn your right foot out 90 degrees and the left foot in 15 degrees.
- Bend the right knee until the thigh is parallel to the floor.
- Place the right hand behind the right foot.
- Elongate the ribs and revolve the right side of the body forward.
- Stretch the left arm over the head (**Figure 6-8**).
- Repeat the asana on the other side.

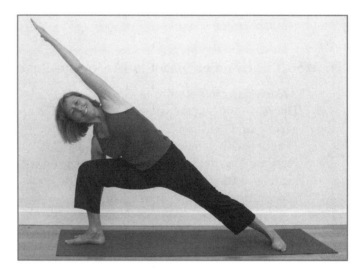

Figure 6-8

Drishti

The gaze can be upward toward the extended arm, forward, or to the floor by the bent knee.

Alignment Cues

- Fully root both feet. Pay special attention to the baby toe side of the back foot.
- Track the bent knee over the second and third toes and press the thigh open.

- Keep the torso from leaning forward or back. Maintain a one-dimensional plane.
- Feel a line of energy from the baby toe of the straight leg to the fingers of the extended arm.
- Revolve the chest and torso upward.

Benefits

This pose will:

- Strengthen and stretch the legs and back
- Increase flexibility in the hips and shoulders
- Energize the digestive system
- Stretch the groin
- Tone the waist and abdominal muscles
- Build stamina

Modifications or Ways to Make the Pose Work for You!

- Place the right forearm on the thigh with the palm facing upward (**Figure 6-9**).

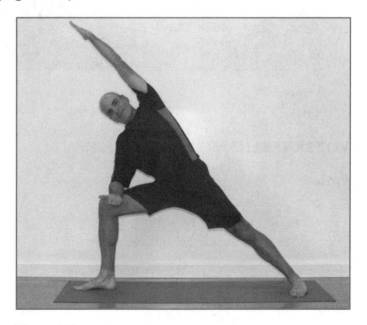

Figure 6-9

- Wrap the top arm around the spine and catch the thigh of the bent knee. Roll the top shoulder and chest open.
- Place the right hand on a block that is in front or behind the right foot.
- Place the right hand on the floor in front of the right foot.
- For the more advanced student, try Warrior Interlock. Reach the right arm under the thigh. Reach the left arm up and over the back. The right hand will then clasp the left wrist (**Figure 6-10**).

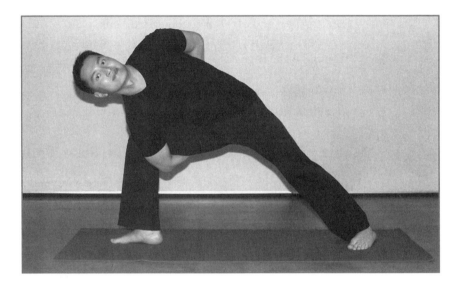

Figure 6-10

PARSVOTTANASANA: PYRAMID POSE

Description

- Start in Tadasana.
- Step the left foot back 3 to 3½ feet.
- Place the hands behind the back and hold the elbows with the hands.
- Lengthen and energize the legs, keeping them straight.
- Lift and arch the chest upward.

- Hinge the torso forward from the hip joint while lengthening the entire spine from the tailbone to the top of the head (**Figure 6-11A**).
- Fold forward until the chin touches the shin (**Figure 6-11B**).
- Repeat the asana on the other side.

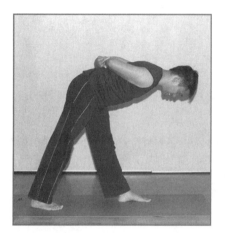

Figure 6-11A

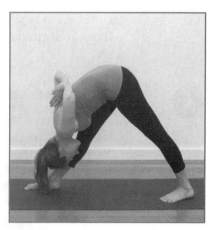

Figure 6-11B

Drishti

The gaze should be toward the front leg.

Alignment Cues

- Align the front heel with the back heel.
- The back foot is slightly turned out. The front foot is facing directly forward.
- Keep the back leg strong and straight.
- To square the hips, rotate the left hip bone forward and the right hip bone back.
- Turn both shoulders forward so they are directly above the hips.
- When bending forward, lengthen the torso away from the hip joint.
- When folded forward, lift the sit bones up and back.

Benefits

This pose will:

- Stretch the legs, back, and shoulders
- Increase hip, shoulder, and wrist joint flexibility
- Strengthen the legs
- Develop balance
- Improve stamina

Modifications or Ways to Make the Pose Work for You!

- Bend the front knee as needed.
- Interlace the fingers behind the back, place palms in reverse Namaste, or, for extra support, place hands on the floor by the front foot.
- Pose can start with arms stretched overhead, palms together, and thumbs crossing.

Yoga Science

The health-related aspects of physical fitness—defined as muscular strength and endurance, general flexibility, cardiopulmonary endurance, and body composition as well as pulmonary function—were evaluated in a study of volunteers before and after eight weeks of yoga practice (Raub, 2002). The study was composed of people ages 18 to 27. Significant increases were found in all the components of fitness except for body composition.

Student Testimonial

"Since I began practicing yoga, I have noticed improved coordination and concentration in other daily activities. Even painting the inside of my house was easier."

UTKATASANA: CHAIR POSE

Description

- Start in Tadasana.
- Hinge from the hip joint so the tailbone moves backward and downward.
- Bend your knees as though you were sitting in a chair and the thighs form a right angle with your shins.
- Squeeze your ankles, knees, and thighs together.
- Float the arms upward until the palms are facing each other overhead (**Figure 6–12**).

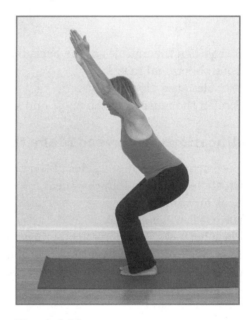

Figure 6-12

Drishti

Gaze should be upward or forward.

Alignment Cues

- Ground the four corners of the feet evenly into floor.
- Engage the inner thigh muscles fully by squeezing the knees together.

- Imagine sitting in a chair.
- Bend the knees as much as possible, keeping the heels on the ground.
- Keep most of the weight on the heels.
- Feel as if the arms are hanging from a tree and your tailbone is pulling toward the floor.
- Draw the shoulder blades down the back.
- Draw the chin toward the throat so the neck stays long if looking forward.

Benefits

This pose will:

- Strengthen the muscles of the back, buttocks, legs, and ankles
- Tone abdominal muscles
- Stimulate the digestive system
- Stretch the muscles of the chest and shoulders

Modifications or Ways to Make the Pose Work for You!

- Keep arms down by the sides of the body or straight forward.
- Create less of a bend in the knees.
- Look forward.
- Have feet wider apart.
- Place buttocks and spine flat against the wall. Have the feet about 18 inches from wall. Bend the knees until the thighs are parallel to the wall and shins are directly over the ankles. The arms can be stretched parallel to the floor or hands can be in Namaste.

PARIVRTTA TRIKONASANA: REVOLVING TRIANGLE POSE

Description

- Start in Tadasana
- Step the left foot back 3 to 3½ feet.
- Place the hands on the waist.
- Lengthen and energize the legs, keeping them straight.
- Lift and arch the chest upward.
- Hinge the torso forward from the hip joint while lengthening the entire spine from the tailbone to the top of the head.

- Keep the spine parallel to the floor and place the left hand either on the shin, by the big toe, or on the baby toe side of the right foot.
- Stretch the right arm upward so that the arms make a straight line (**Figure 6-13**).
- Repeat the asana on the other side.

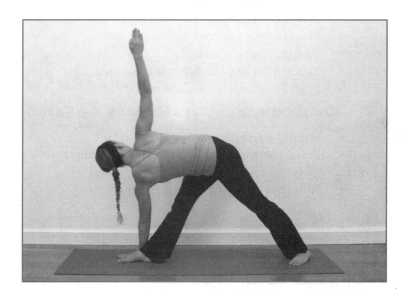

Figure 6-13

Drishti

The gaze is upward toward the top hand, neutral, or downward at the floor.

Alignment Cues

- Ground the four corners of the feet.
- Lift the knee caps to activate the quadriceps.
- Square the hips by revolving the right hip back and the left hip forward.
- Lengthen the waist equally on both sides.
- Lengthen the spine and lift the sternum as you hinge forward.
- Rotate the torso upward as you roll the right shoulder back.
- Energize the arms, while creating a straight line from fingertip to fingertip.

Benefits

This pose will:

*   Relieve lower back discomfort
*   Increase flexibility in the hips
*   Strengthen the legs
*   Massage the internal organs
*   Energize the entire body
*   Stimulate right-left brain coordination

Modifications or Ways to Make the Pose Work for You!

*   Bend the front knee.
*   Place the hand on a block either to the inside or outside of the foot.
*   Keep the extended arm on the hip.

PRASARITA PADOTTANASANA: EXTENDED LEG FORWARD BEND POSE

Description

*   Start in Tadasana.
*   Jump or step at least 4 feet apart.
*   Place hands on the waist.
*   Hinge from the hip joints and bend until the spine is parallel to floor.
*   Place hands on the floor in line with the arches of the feet. The fingertips face forward.
*   Bend the elbows backward.
*   Rest the top of the head on the floor (**Figure 6-14**).

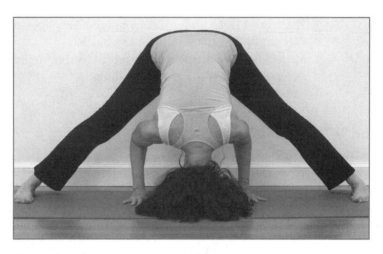

Figure 6-14

Drishti

The gaze is toward the third eye or the floor.

Alignment Cues

- Ground the four corners of the feet.
- Lift the kneecaps to keep the legs straight.
- Internally rotate the thighs as you hinge forward.
- Stretch the spine to create length from the tailbone to the crown of the head.
- Keep the hips in line with the ankles when you are folded forward.
- Tuck the head under so that the top of the head reaches the floor.

Benefits

This pose will:

- Strengthen the legs and ankles
- Increase flexibility in the hamstrings and lower back
- Calm the mind and nerves

Modifications or Ways to Make the Pose Work for You!

- Take legs wider to get the head to the floor.
- Bend the knees as necessary.

- Place two blocks under the shoulders. Keep the spine parallel to the floor and place the hands on the blocks.
- More advanced students can interlace the fingers behind the back and reach palms toward the ceiling.

MALASANA: BASIC SQUAT POSE

Description

- Start in Tadasana with the feet about 8 inches apart and the hands in Namaste.
- Energetically root through the four corners of the feet.
- Open the chest and roll the shoulder blades down the back.
- Slowly bend the knees until the knees are fully flexed.
- Press the elbows to the insides of the thighs to lift the chest and lengthen the spine (**Figure 6-15**).

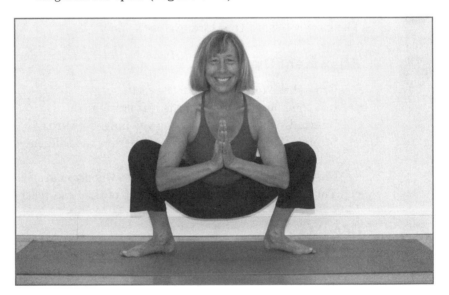

Figure 6-15

 Drishti

The gaze is straight ahead or eyes are closed.

Alignment Cues

- Keep the heels firmly planted on the ground.
- Release the tailbone to the floor without rolling the knees inward.
- Keep the spine long and open.
- Roll the armpits and chest forward.

 ## Benefits

This pose will:

- Strengthen the feet and ankles
- Open the hips
- Strengthen the spine
- Improve balance and poise
- Prepare one for childbirth

 ## Modifications or How to Make the Pose Work for You!

- Have the feet farther apart to make the pose easier.
- Place the heels on a folded blanket if heels cannot stay flat on the ground (**Figure 6–16**).
- Use a wall behind the lower back for stability and alignment.

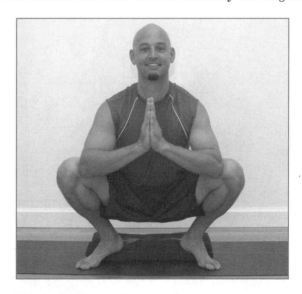

Figure 6-16

STUDY QUESTIONS

1. Name three ways in which the standing poses benefit the body.
2. Name three guidelines for performing standing poses.
3. How is the alignment of Tadasana utilized in the other standing poses?
4. Describe three alignment cues for Virabhadrasana II.
5. Describe two modifications for Utkatasana.

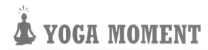 # YOGA MOMENT

Practice Utthita Parsvakonasana (Side Angle Bend) on both sides with and then without a block. Record your observations.

CHAPTER SEVEN

Balance Poses

Be Steady and Stable

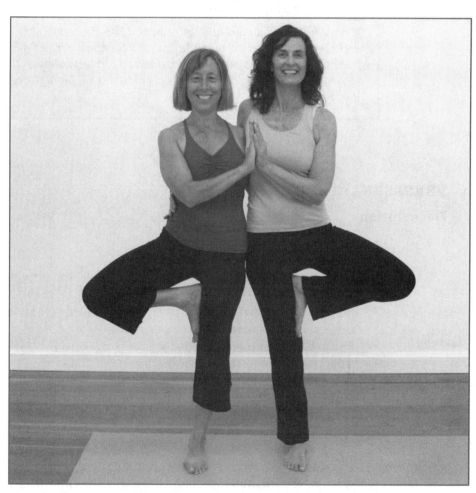

Praise and blame, gain and loss, pleasure and sorrow, come and go like the wind. To be happy, rest like a giant tree, in the midst of them all.

— **Buddha**

The balance poses require focus (find a drishti point), correct alignment (find Tadasana), coordination, flexibility, and strength. The body integrates in harmony and grace when practicing balance.

> " ,, **Student Testimonial**
>
> *"I have always disliked hiking because I hated crossing creeks and climbing rocks for fear of losing my balance. Since I have begun practicing yoga my balance has improved so much that rather than dreading those moments on the trail, I look forward to these challenges!"*

VRKSASANA: TREE POSE

Description

- Start in Tadasana.
- Shift the weight to the right foot.
- Use your left hand to bring your left foot to the inner right thigh or groin.
- Equally press the right inner thigh to the left sole of the foot.
- Bring the hands together to prayer pose.
- Press the palms together equally.
- Bring the arms to the top of the head and then extend the arms above the head (**Figure 7-1**).
- Maintain balance.
- Repeat pose on the other leg.

Drishti

The gaze is forward, and eventually the gaze goes upward.

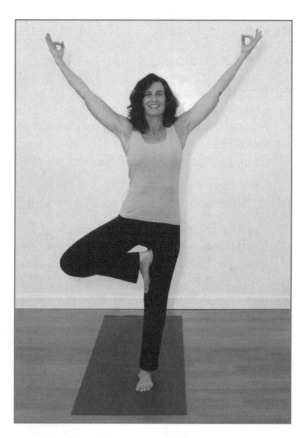

Figure 7-1

Alignment Cues

- Push firmly into the four corners of the foot; focus on keeping the big toe rooted.
- Lift the kneecap of the standing leg to engage the quadriceps.
- Make sure both hips are pointed forward and are on the same plane.
- Open the knee of the bent leg as far to the side as possible.
- Extend the tailbone downward toward the floor and the crown of the head upward, creating length and extension in the spine.
- Lift the sides of the body equally without pushing the ribs outward.
- Move the shoulder blades down the back.
- Allow the strength of the extended arms to lengthen the pose.

Benefits

This pose will:

- Improve balance
- Lengthen the spine
- Strengthen the feet, ankles, calves, and thighs
- Open the hips
- Calm the mind and build concentration

Modifications or Ways to Make the Pose Work for You!

- Practice the pose against a wall.
- Keep the hands in prayer pose by the chest (**Figure 7-2**).
- Practice the pose with the foot by the ankle.

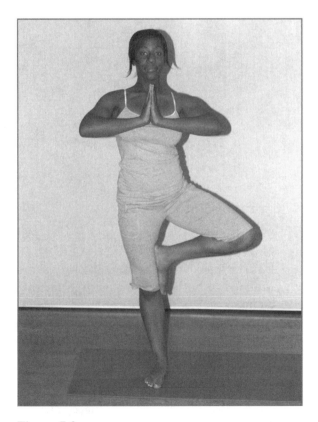

Figure 7-2

GARUDASANA: EAGLE POSE

Description

- Start in Tadasana.
- Bring the right arm to a right angle in front of the body with the palm facing inward and the fingers pointing upward.
- Cross the left elbow underneath the right arm and bring the palms of the hands together.
- Bend both knees to chair pose.
- Shift the weight to the right leg and hook the left foot behind the right calf, squeezing both legs together (**Figure 7-3**).
- Maintain balance.
- Repeat on the other side.

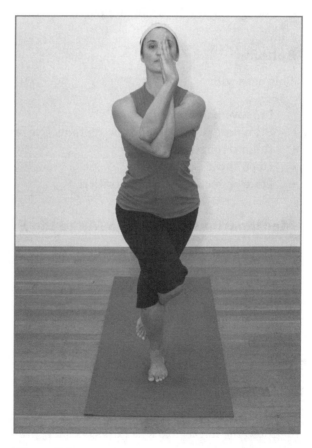

Figure 7-3

Drishti

The gaze is forward.

Alignment Cues

- Spread the toes of the standing leg.
- Keep both hips facing forward and on a parallel plane.
- Squeeze the legs tightly together.
- Squeeze the arms together.
- Raise the elbows to shoulder level.
- Draw the shoulder blades down the back.
- Bend the supporting knee as much as possible, keeping the knee in line with the second and third toes.
- Keep the chin drawn in and parallel to the floor.

Benefits

This pose will:

- Improve balance
- Stimulate digestion and the reproductive organs
- Build strength in the legs
- Open the shoulders
- Develop focus and concentration

Modifications or Ways to Make the Pose Work for You!

- Practice the leg position and arm position separately.
- Practice against a wall.
- Cross the leg at the ankle joint, or place the ankle on the supporting thigh.

ALANASANA: CRESCENT LUNGE POSE

Description

- Start in Uttanasana (Forward Bend).
- Step the left leg back as far as possible, pressing into the ball of the foot.

- Palms are flat on the floor by the right ankle.
- Lengthen the torso over the right thigh.
- Lift the torso until the shoulders are over the hips.
- Place the hands on the buttocks and push the hips forward.
- Open the chest as the arms stretch overhead.
- Stretch the arms upward and then clasp the hands with the index fingers extended (**Figure 7-4**).

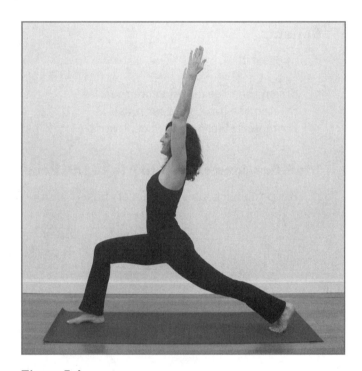

Figure 7-4

Drishti

The gaze is upward toward the fingertips or straight ahead.

Alignment Cues

- Step far enough back so that the palms are flat on the floor by the front ankle.
- Push fully through the back heel.

- Lift the back of the knee upward.
- Fully extend the back leg and lift the hamstrings upward.
- Align the front knee exactly over the ankle.
- Press the hips forward and drop the tailbone.
- Fully engage the abdominals.
- Lift and open the chest.
- With the arms extended, draw the shoulder blades down the back.

 ## Benefits

This pose will:

- Strengthen the leg and core muscles
- Stretch the hip and chest muscles
- Promote balance and concentration

 ## Modifications or How to Make the Pose Work for You!

- Keep the back knee and top of the foot on the floor (**Figure 7-5**).

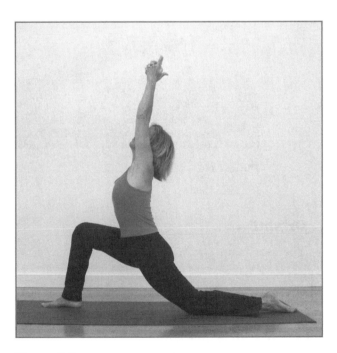

Figure 7-5

- Use a blanket under the back knee.
- Keep the hands unclasped and the arms shoulder distance apart.
- Use blocks for the hands next to the front ankle.

ARDHA CHANDRASANA: HALF MOON POSE

Description

- Start in Utthita Trikonasana (Triangle pose) with the right foot at 90 degrees and the left foot turned inward at 15 degrees.
- Take your left hand to the left hip and turn the gaze to the right big toe.
- Bend the right knee and place the right hand on the floor (or a block) 8 to 10 inches in front of the baby toe side of the foot.
- Shift the weight onto the right leg and straighten the leg.
- Extend the left leg parallel to the floor and flex the left toes.
- Extend the left arm upward, directly above the shoulder (**Figure 7-6**).

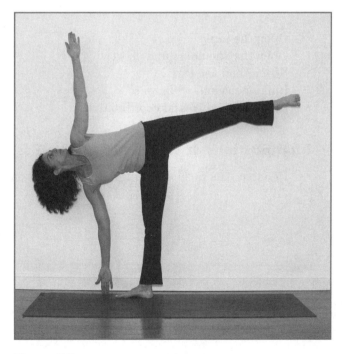

Figure 7-6

Drishti

The gaze in this pose begins at the floor with focus on the standing foot. When the balance is achieved, the gaze turns forward. Eventually, the gaze goes upward toward the thumb of the lifted hand.

Alignment Cues

- Keep the standing leg fully extended.
- Create a straight line between the two extended arms.
- Stack the hips directly on top of each other.
- Flatten the entire torso against an imaginary wall.
- Find length from the navel through the crown of the head.
- Place the supporting hand directly under the shoulder.
- Completely straighten the lifted leg, making sure the knee faces forward.

Benefits

This pose will:

- Open the hips
- Open the shoulders and chest
- Strengthen the legs
- Build focus and willpower
- Improve balance and coordination

Modifications or Ways to Make the Pose Work for You!

- Practice this pose standing against a wall using a block (**Figure 7-7**).

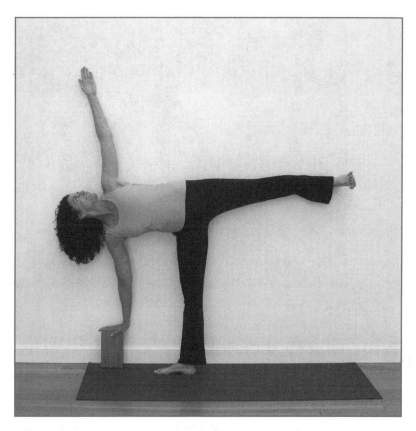

Figure 7-7

VIRABHADRASANA III: WARRIOR III POSE
Description

- Start in Tadasana with the hands in prayer pose.
- Step the right foot forward about 2 feet. Keep the right knee bent.
- Hinge from the hip joint until the spine is parallel to the floor.
- Lift the left leg directly behind you, parallel to the floor.
- When you achieve balance, straighten the supporting leg and extend the arms directly overhead (**Figure 7-8**).

 ### Drishti

Gaze straight ahead or at the floor.

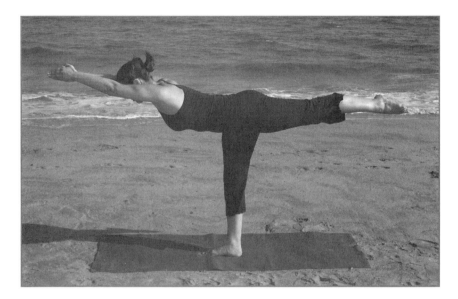

Figure 7-8

Alignment Cues

- Keep both hips facing the floor and align them in Tadasana.
- Fully engage the muscles on both legs.
- Keep the knee of the lifted leg facing the floor.
- Lengthen the torso from the crown of the head to the heel of the extended leg.

Benefits

This pose will:

- Build strength in the legs and torso
- Improve balance and focus
- Tone abdominal muscles
- Develop willpower and stimulate the mind

Modifications or How to Make the Pose Work for You!

- Use a wall or a chair for balance.
- Keep the standing leg slightly bent.
- Keep the hands in prayer pose.

- Position the arms out to the sides like an airplane or keep the hands by the side of the body (**Figure 7-9**).

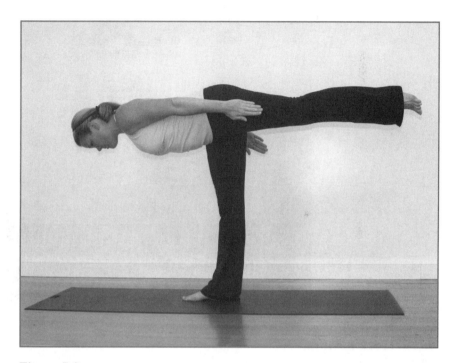

Figure 7-9

NATARAJASANA: DANCER'S POSE

Description

- Start in Tadasana.
- Bend the left knee back toward the buttocks.
- Hold the inside of the left foot with the left hand.
- Extend the right arm directly upward.
- Hinge from the hip joint and lift the left leg upward (**Figure 7-10**).
- Repeat the pose on the other leg.

 Drishti

The gaze is toward the extended fingertips.

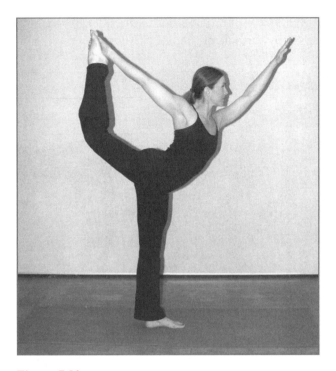

Figure 7-10

Alignment Cues

- Keep the hips level as in Tadasana.
- The knee of the extended leg is facing down toward the floor.
- Open the chest creating a backbend.
- Create as much distance between the hip bones and chest as possible.
- Fully engage the muscles of the standing leg.
- Feel a stretch in both directions.

Benefits

This pose will:

- Develop flexibility in the chest and shoulders
- Strengthen the legs and spinal muscles
- Increase balance and coordination
- Develop grace

Modifications or Ways to Make the Pose Work for You!

- Hold a strap, which has been looped around the lifted foot or ankle (**Figure 7–11**).
- Use a wall for balance.
- Hold the ankle without lifting the leg upward.

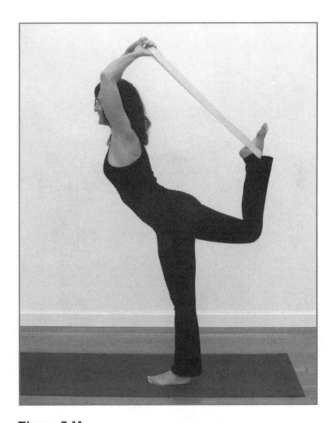

Figure 7-11

UTTHITA HASTA PADANGUSTASANA: EXTENDED HAND TO TOE POSE

Description

- Start in Tadasana.
- Bend your right knee, bring your right hand to the inside of the leg, and grab the inside of the big toe with the first two fingers.

- Place the left hand on the left hip and extend the right leg forward.
- Rotate the right leg outward and carry it to the side.
- Extend the left arm to the side and turn the head toward the left hand (**Figure 7-12**).
- Repeat this pose on the other leg.

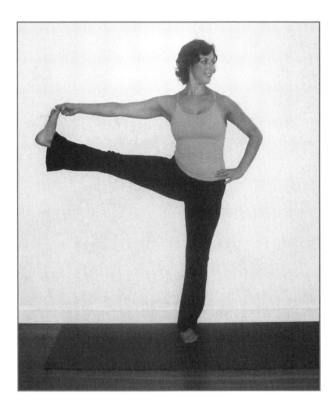

Figure 7-12

Drishti

Gaze forward when the leg is extended forward and gaze at the extended arm when the leg is to the side.

Alignment Cues

- Keep both hips facing forward with special attention to the hip of the extended leg.
- Open the chest.
- Draw the shoulder blades down the back.
- Lift through the crown of the head.
- Keep the muscles of the standing leg fully engaged.
- Keep the lifted leg straight.
- Keep the toes of the standing leg facing forward.

Benefits

This pose will:

- Stretch the hamstrings
- Strengthen the legs and abdominal muscles
- Develop balance, flexibility, and focus

Modifications or Making the Pose Work for You!

- Use a strap to hold the leg (**Figure 7–13**).
- Extend the leg forward without holding on to it.
- Place the back against a wall for balance.
- Place the leg on a chair, fitness ball, or ballet barre.
- Standing with the back against a wall, let a partner slowly carry the lifted leg to the side.

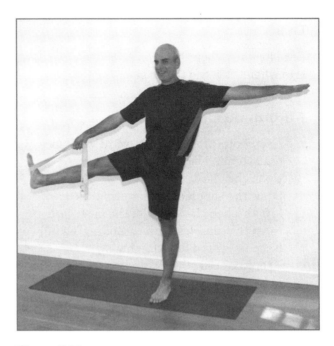

Figure 7-13

STUDY QUESTIONS

1. What elements are needed when practicing balance poses?
2. Pretend you are a yoga instructor and guide a student into Eagle pose using correct alignment cues.
3. What balance poses can be modified by using a belt? By using a block?
4. Describe three alignment cues for Virabhadrasana III.
5. Describe three modifications for Vrksasana.

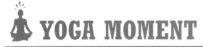

YOGA MOMENT

Stand in Tadasana and rise onto the balls of your feet. Practice this with the eyes closed. Record your observations.

CHAPTER EIGHT

Arm-Supported Poses

"May the Force Be With You"

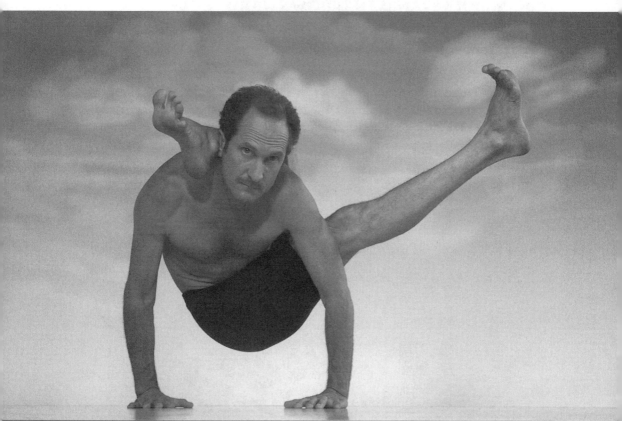

This yoga should be practiced with firm determination and perseverance, without mental reservation or doubts.

— **The Bhagavad Gita**

These asanas require arm, core, and leg strength and create a balance and harmony between the arm and leg muscles by fully engaging the muscles and drawing them to the bone. Be aware of the lines of energy within these arm-supported poses to create radiance and strength.

ADHO MUKHA SVANASANA: DOWNWARD FACING DOG POSE

Description

- Start on all fours with the hands under the shoulders and the knees under the hips.
- Move the hands about one foot in front of the shoulders.
- Tuck the toes under and straighten the legs (**Figure 8-1**).

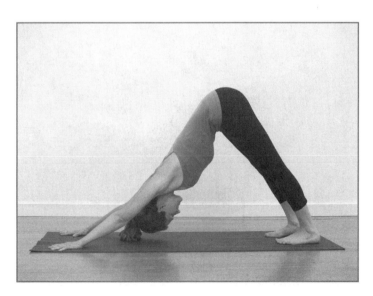

Figure 8-1

Drishti

The gaze is downward toward the floor or between the big toes.

Alignment Cues

- Press the palms evenly into the ground and extend through all 10 finger pads.
- The middle fingers stretch forward and the thumbs stretch toward each other.
- Activate the arm muscles as the elbows draw toward each other, which broadens the upper back.
- Draw the shoulder blades down the back.
- Press the chest toward the thighs and belly.
- Lift and spread the sit bones upward.
- Create two straight legs by engaging the quadriceps. Let the legs work strongly.
- Sink the heels into the floor.
- Draw the thighbones back toward the hamstrings and the shinbones back toward the calves.
- Draw the inner thighs backward.
- Release the head to eliminate any tension in the neck.

Benefits

This pose will:

- Energize the entire body
- Stretch and strengthen the entire body
- Build endurance
- Create more shoulder flexibility
- Prepare the arms for more advanced inversions

Modifications or How to Make the Pose Work for You!

- Walk the Dog: Bend the right knee and drop the left heel to the ground. Repeat slowly on the other side.

- Puppy pose: Bring both feet together and bend both knees. Lift the sit bones higher and lengthen the sides of the body (**Figure 8-2**).
- Dolphin pose: Start on the hands and elbows with the hands clasped or flat on the ground. Tuck the toes under and straighten the legs.

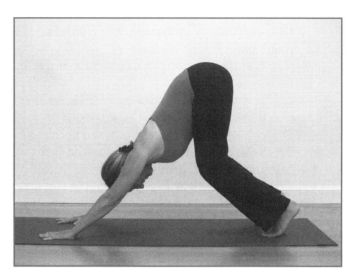

Figure 8-2

URDHVA MUKHA SVANASANA: UPWARD FACING DOG POSE

Description

- Lie flat on your stomach.
- Fully engage the leg muscles with the tops of the feet pressing into the floor.
- Place the palms under the shoulders with the fingers spread wide.
- Draw the chest forward while squeezing the elbows into the sides of the body.
- As you straighten the elbows, lift the torso off the ground until only the tops of the feet contact the floor (**Figure 8-3A** and **Figure 8-3B**).

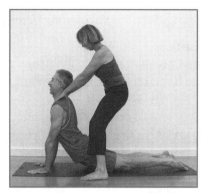 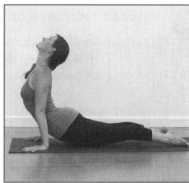

Figure 8-3A   **Figure 8-3B**

Drishti

The gaze is forward or toward the third eye.

Alignment Cues

- Press the tops of the feet firmly into the floor with the toes spread.
- Rotate the thighs inward.
- Fully engage the buttocks muscles.
- Lengthen both sides of the body equally.
- Draw the shoulder blades down the back.
- Draw the underneath part of the armpits forward to open the chest.
- Keep the chin parallel to the floor and the back of the neck long.
- Feel the crown of the head reaching upward.

Benefits

This pose will:

- Strengthen the spine, legs, and arms
- Open the chest
- Promote deep breathing and improve lung capacity
- Increase spinal flexibility
- Stretch the abdominals and hip flexors
- Stimulate the nervous system

Modifications or How to Make the Pose Work for You!

* Keep the thighs on the floor.
* Curl the toes under and press them into the floor.
* Place blocks under the hands to lessen the curve of the spine.

UTTHITA CHATURANGA DANDASANA: PLANK POSE

Description

* Start in the standard push-up position, with the hands spread wide under the shoulders, legs extended directly back, and the toes tucked
* Lengthen the upper body through the crown of the head.
* Lengthen the lower body through the heels (**Figure 8-4**).

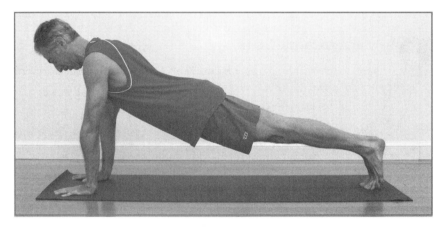

Figure 8-4

Drishti

The gaze is on the floor directly under the eyes.

Alignment Cues

* Keep the body strong and straight like a redwood board.
* Feel two lines of energy, from the belly to the crown of the head and from the belly out through the heels.
* Draw the navel toward the spine.

- Draw the shoulder blades down the back.
- Press the hip bones toward the floor.
- Fully engage the legs and arms by drawing the muscles toward the bones.
- Press firmly through the heels to fully activate the leg muscles.
- The hands are directly under the shoulders.
- The eye of the elbows face forward.
- Keep the feet together.

Benefits

This pose will:

- Strengthen the arms and legs
- Build core strength
- Energize the entire body
- Develop willpower

Modifications or How to Make the Pose Work for You!

- Place the knees on the floor (**Figure 8-5**).
- For an additional challenge, lift one leg at a time off the floor.
- Place the forearms on the floor.

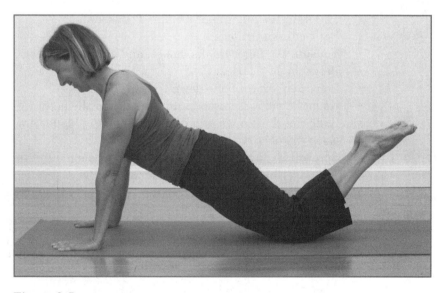

Figure 8-5

CHATURANGA DANDASANA: LOW PLANK POSE

Description

- Start in Plank pose.
- With the body parallel to the floor, lower down until the upper arms are parallel to the floor.
- Maintain the body 2 to 3 inches from the floor (**Figure 8–6**).

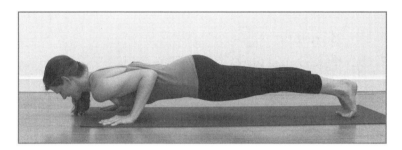

Figure 8-6

Drishti

The gaze is on the floor or forward.

Alignment Cues

- Maintain the alignment used in Tadasana.
- Fully engage the legs.
- Squeeze the inner thighs, knees, and ankles together.
- Press the heels back.
- Lengthen the tailbone down toward the heels.
- Keep the elbows pressed into the sides of the body.
- Keep the chest open and draw the shoulder blades down the back.
- Keep the back of the neck long.
- Spread the fingers wide and press the whole hand into the floor.

Benefits

This pose will:

- Strengthen the arms, legs, wrists, buttocks, and shoulders
- Develop core strength
- Energize the entire body

Modifications or Ways to Make the Pose Work for You!

- Keep the knees on the floor.
- Adjust the hand position forward or wider apart to make the pose easier on the wrists.

PURVOTTANASANA: UPWARD PLANK POSE

Description

- Start in Dandasana (see Chapter 9) with the hands behind the hips.
- Bend your knees, rooting the four corners of the feet into the floor.
- Keep the feet parallel and hip distance apart.
- Lift the hips to the ceiling, creating a table top with your torso.
- Straighten and extend the legs, pointing the toes and keeping the heels on the floor.
- Fully engage the buttocks muscle and lift up.
- Slowly lift the chin upward and stretch the neck (**Figure 8-7**).

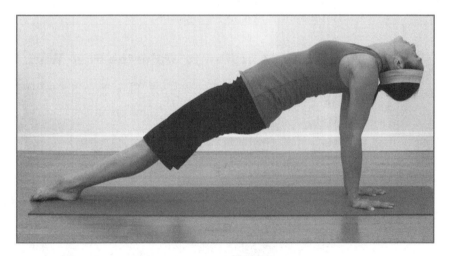

Figure 8-7

Drishti

The gaze is upward.

Alignment Cues

- Extend fully through the toes.
- Internally rotate the thighs.
- Fully extend and activate the legs.
- Press the hip bones toward the ceiling.
- Lengthen both sides of the body.
- Squeeze the shoulder blades together to open the chest.
- Create as much distance between the ears and shoulders as possible.
- Draw the elbows in toward the sides of the body.
- Lengthen through the sides of the throat.
- Do not strain the neck.

Benefits

This pose will:

- Strengthen the arms, wrists, buttocks, legs, and ankles
- Energize the body
- Open the chest and throat
- Build endurance and willpower

Modifications or How to Make the Pose Work for You!

- Keep the knees bent in the table top position (**Figure 8-8**).
- Point the fingers away from the feet.
- Rest the chin by the chest.

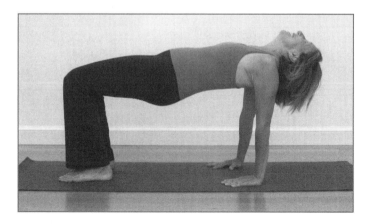

Figure 8-8

VASISTHASANA: SAGE POSE (ONE ARM PLANK POSE)

Description

- Start in Plank pose.
- Move the left hand under the center of the chest.
- Roll to the outside of the left foot.
- Place the right leg directly on top of the left leg with the feet flexed.
- Extend the right arm to the ceiling.
- Turn the head to look at the right hand (**Figure 8-9**).
- Repeat on the other side.

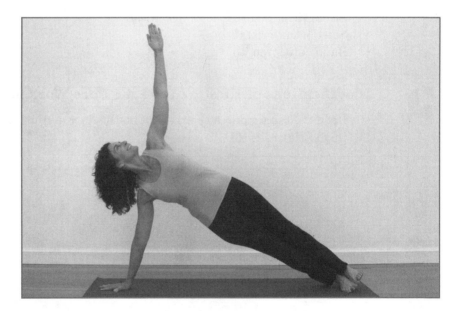

Figure 8-9

Drishti

The gaze is upward toward the lifted hand or straight ahead.

Alignment Cues

- The hand on the ground is directly under the shoulder.
- Press the palms and fingers into the floor.
- Keep both sides of the body fully lifted.

- Stretch through the crown of the head and through the soles of the feet.
- Fully engage the core muscles.
- Draw the tailbone down toward the feet.
- Draw the navel toward the spine.
- Create a straight line between both arms.

 ## Benefits

This pose will:

- Improve balance
- Strengthen the arms, legs, and wrists
- Stretch the wrists
- Build core strength

 ## Modifications or How to Make the Pose Work for You!

- Bend the top leg and place the foot on the floor in front of the lower thigh (**Figure 8-10**).

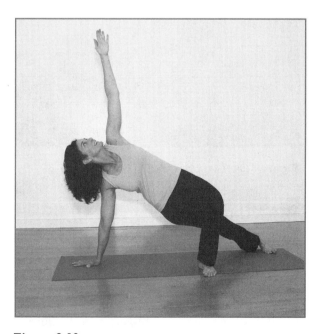

Figure 8-10

- Extend the top arm overhead.
- Lift the top leg up.
- Put the top leg in Tree pose.
- Place the bottom knee on the floor, keeping all parts of the body that are touching the floor in a straight line (**Figure 8-11**).

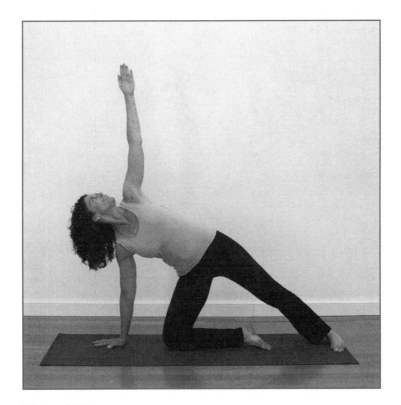

Figure 8-11

STUDY QUESTIONS

1. What is the value of practicing arm-supported asanas?
2. How is the alignment of Tadasana utilized in Plank pose?
3. How many lines of energy are in Downward Facing Dog pose? Where are those lines of energy?
4. Describe three modifications for Vasisthasana.
5. Describe three alignment cues for Urdhva Mukha Svanasana.

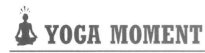

YOGA MOMENT

Practice Plank pose for twenty seconds. Practice Plank pose for thirty seconds. Practice Plank pose for one minute. Were you able to keep your breath fluid and free? Were you strong yet relaxed? Record your observations.

CHAPTER NINE

Sitting and Kneeling Poses

Find Your Center

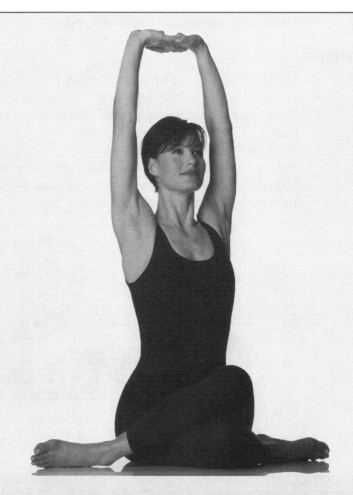

Courage is what it takes to stand up and speak.
Courage is also what it takes to sit down and listen.

— **Winston Churchill**

Student Testimonial

"I never realized the focus and attention it takes just to sit up straight until I started yoga. Now I can work at the computer for hours without lower back pain or neck and shoulder tension."

DANDASANA: STAFF POSE

This pose is the foundation for all sitting poses.

Description

- Sit on the yoga mat with legs extended straight in front of you.
- Position the legs so the inner thighs and ankles touch.
- Balance on your sit bones by moving the fleshy part of the buttocks back.
- Place the hands next to the hips.
- Push down through the palms all the way through the fingertips to extend the spine and open the chest (**Figure 9-1**).
- Press the chest through the armpits.

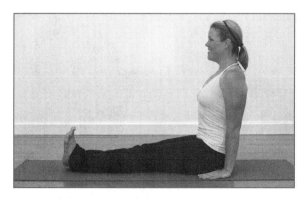

Figure 9-1

Drishti

The gaze is forward.

Alignment Cues

- As in Tadasana, the ears are directly above the shoulders, and the shoulders are directly above the hips.
- Float the crown of the head toward the ceiling.
- Draw the shoulder blades down the back while lifting and opening the chest.
- Move the sacrum forward and upward.
- The kneecaps face upward and the quadriceps are fully engaged.
- Extend fully through the four corners of the feet.

Benefits

This pose will:

- Strengthen the spine
- Tone the abdominal muscles
- Encourage proper alignment

Modifications or How to Make the Pose Work for You!

- Sit on one or two folded blankets to elevate the hips (**Figure 9-2**).
- If the arms are long, take the hands behind the hips.
- To increase the openness of the chest, turn the hands back so fingers face away from the body.
- Practice this posture sitting against a wall.

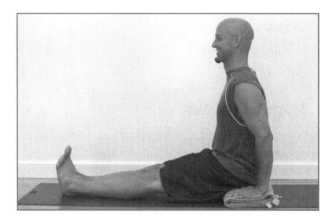

Figure 9-2

PASCHIMOTTANASANA: SEATED FORWARD BEND POSE
Description

- Start in Dandasana.
- Lift the arms over the head.
- Hinge forward from the hips, keeping the arms extended.
- Using the index and middle fingers, hold the inside of the big toes.
- Fold the torso and head over the legs (**Figure 9-3**).

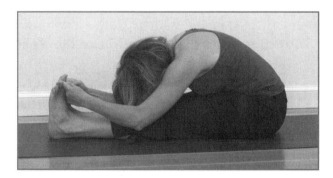

Figure 9-3

Drishti

Gaze forward in Dandasana and gaze toward the shins when folded over the legs.

Alignment Cues

- Fully engage the legs.
- Enliven the four corners of the feet.
- Draw the shoulder blades down the back to lift and open the chest.
- With the arms extended, lengthen the sides of the body equally.
- Draw the ribcage toward the spine.
- While hinging forward, continually draw the lower back in and keep the chest lifted and open.
- Release the head fully toward the knees.

Benefits

This pose will:

- Stretch the hamstrings and the back
- Tone the legs and abdominals
- Quiet the mind and relax the nervous system

Modifications or How to Make the Pose Work for You!

- Sit on one or two folded blankets.
- Hold a strap that has been looped around the feet.
- To work deeper into the pose, hold on to the sides of the feet and draw the elbows to the floor.

JANUSHIRASANA: HEAD TO KNEE POSE

Description

- Start in Dandasana.
- Bend the right leg and place the right foot against the left upper thigh.
- Push down through the left hand and lengthen the spine.
- Reach the right hand to the baby toe side of the left foot to revolve the torso to the left.
- Once the torso is rotated, lift the arms overhead.
- Hinge forward and bring the forehead to the knee and the hands to the foot (**Figure 9-4**).
- Repeat on the other side.

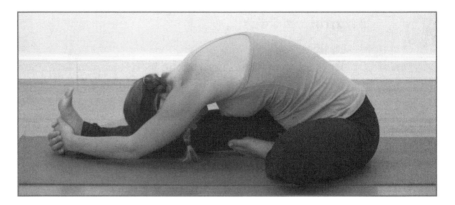

Figure 9-4

Drishti

The gaze is forward in Dandasana and toward the extended shin when folded forward.

Alignment Cues

- Lengthen and engage the extended leg to give stability to the pose.
- Keep the chest lifted and open throughout the entire pose.
- Think of reaching the ribcage over the thighs when bending forward.
- Release the forehead to the knee.

Benefits

This pose will:

- Stretch the legs, hips, and back
- Tone the abdominal muscles
- Expand the lungs and chest
- Calm the mind and reduce stress

Modifications or Ways to Make the Pose Work for You!

- Sit on one or two folded blankets.
- Use a strap around the extended foot.

- Hold the extended foot with the opposite hand and reach the other arm back, revolving the chest and shoulder.

SUKHASANA: EASY POSE

Description

- Sit in Dandasana, bend the knees, and cross the legs at the shins.
- Take the hands by the hips and press into the floor.
- Elongate the torso and stretch the crown of the head upward.
- Place the palms of the hands on the knees (**Figure 9-5**).

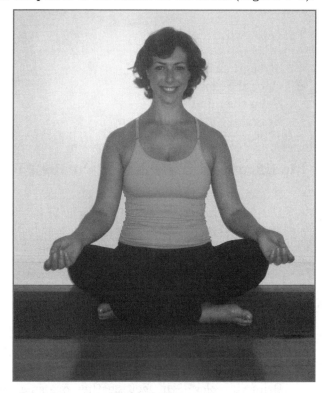

Figure 9-5

 ### Drishti

The gaze is forward.

Alignment Cues

- Balance the weight in the sit bones evenly.
- Lengthen both sides of the torso equally.
- Float the crown of the head toward the ceiling.
- Draw the shoulder blades down the back, creating as much space between the ears and shoulders as possible.
- Move the sacrum forward and upward.
- Maintain a long spine and open chest.

Benefits

This pose will:

- Strengthen the back
- Open the hips
- Calm the mind
- Encourage proper alignment

Modifications or Ways to Make the Pose Work for You!

- Sit on one or two folded blankets.
- Use folded blankets under the thighs or knees for support.
- Practice this posture sitting against a wall.

BADDHA KONASANA: BOUND ANGLE POSE

Description

- Start in Dandasana.
- Bend the knees and draw the heels in toward the groin.
- Bring the soles of the feet together, pressing equally.
- Place the hands behind the hips with the fingertips facing backward (**Figure 9-6**).
- Stay in this position until spine and chest are lifted.
- To deepen the pose, grab the feet with your hands and press the spine inward to lift and open the chest.

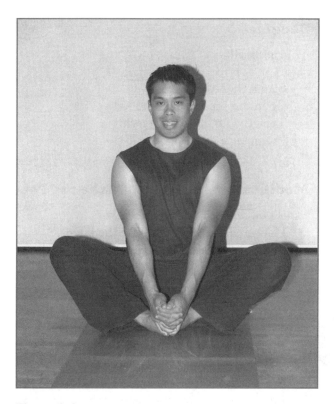

Figure 9-6

Drishti

The gaze is forward.

Alignment Cues

- Create balance and symmetry in the body by evenly distributing the weight in the hips, legs, and feet.
- Draw the shoulder blades down the back.
- Lift and open the chest.
- Lift the crown of the head upward and draw the chin inward.

Benefits

This pose will:

- Strengthen the spine
- Open the hips, groin, and knees
- Tone the abdominal muscles
- Promote proper alignment

 Modifications or How to Make the Pose Work for You!

- Sit on one or two folded blankets.
- Place folded blankets under the knees.
- Support the back by sitting against a wall.

UPAVISTHA KONASANA: WIDE ANGLE SEATED FORWARD BEND POSE

Description

- Start in Baddha Konasana (Bound Angle pose).
- Place the palms of the hands behind the hips and press firmly into the floor to elongate the spine.
- Open the legs outward as wide as possible, keeping the knees facing upward.
- Bring the hands forward to the inside of the thighs while maintaining the length of the torso.
- Hinge forward from the hips, walking the hands forward.
- Grab the big toes with the index and middle fingers while lowering the chest and head toward the floor (**Figure 9-7**).

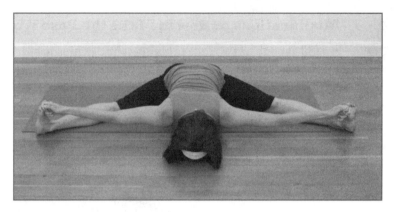

Figure 9-7

Drishti

The gaze is forward when upright and to the ground when the torso is lowered.

Alignment Cues

- Move the fleshy part of the buttocks away to fully sit on the sit bones.
- Rotate the inner thighs forward to keep the knees facing the ceiling.
- Fully engage the legs and feet by pressing the thighs and calves toward the floor.
- Lift and activate the abdominal muscles.
- Lift and open the chest.
- Draw the shoulder blades down the back.
- Move the sacrum and lower back forward.
- Lead with the chest as the torso is lowered to the floor.

Benefits

This pose will:

- Stretch the groin muscles
- Stretch and strengthen the leg muscles
- Lengthen and strengthen the back muscles
- Open the hips and chest
- Promote good posture

Modifications or How to Make the Pose Work for You!

- Sit on one or two folded blankets if the hips are tight.
- Use a blanket under the palms to lift the chest.
- Use two straps around the arches of the feet and grab them with the hands (**Figure 9-8**).

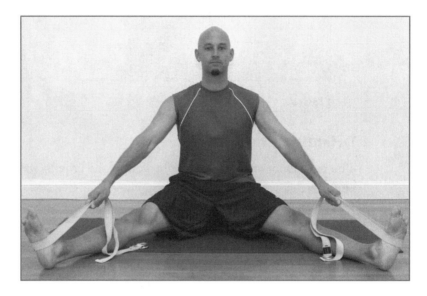

Figure 9-8

- When folding forward, use two folded blankets that stretch from the inner thighs outward and place the forehead on the blankets.
- Use a folding chair with the seat facing your body and a folded blanket over the edge. As you fold forward, let the forehead rest on the chair seat.

NAVASANA: BOAT POSE

Description

- Start in Dandasana.
- Bend the knees with the toes lifted upward, the hands below the kneecaps, and the elbows drawn into the sides.
- Lift the feet off the floor until the lower legs are parallel to the floor.
- Grab the big toes and extend the legs (**Figure 9-9**).

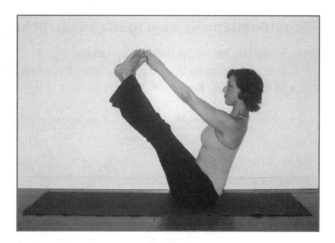

Figure 9-9

Drishti

The gaze is forward at the big toes.

Alignment Cues

- Ground and balance the two sit bones.
- Maintain Tadasana alignment in the torso.
- Fully engage the abdominal muscles.
- Lift and open the chest.
- Fully engage and lengthen the legs.

Benefits

This pose will:

- Build core strength
- Develop balance and focus
- Stretch and strengthen the legs
- Improve posture
- Create calmness

Modifications or How to Make the Pose Work for You!

- Keep the knees in the bent position.
- Use a strap around the soles of the feet throughout the progression of the asana (**Figure 9-10**).

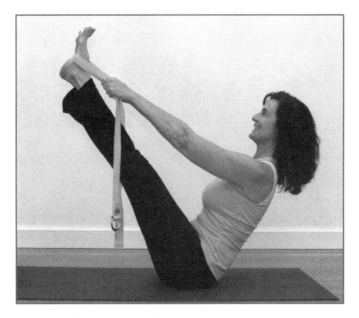

Figure 9-10

ARDHA MATSYENDRASANA: LORD OF THE FISHES POSE (SEATED TWIST)

Description

- Start in Dandasana.
- Bend the right knee and bring the right heel to the outside of the left buttock.
- Bend the left knee, placing the left heel to the outside of the right knee.
- Root through the four corners of the left foot.
- Interlace the hands and place them over the left knee.
- Ground both sit bones and create elegance in this pose by elongating the entire spine.

- Keeping the left hand on the left knee, stretch the right arm skyward.
- Bend the right elbow and place it on the outside of the left knee with the fingers extended upward.
- Place the left hand on the floor behind the tailbone.
- Rotate the torso as far to the left as possible.
- Rotate the head over the left shoulder (**Figure 9-11**).
- Repeat on the other side.

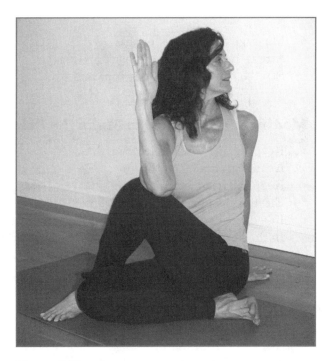

Figure 9-11

Drishti

The gaze is over the back shoulder.

Alignment Cues

- Energize both feet.
- Create balance between both sit bones.
- Draw the shoulder blades down the back.

- Open the chest.
- Reach the crown of the head upward.
- Initiate the twist from the core.
- Move sequentially through the twist.
- Use the inhale to create length and the exhale for the twist.

Benefits

This pose will:

- Massage the internal organs
- Strengthen the neck and back muscles
- Stretch the muscles of the hips and back

Modifications or How to Make the Pose Work for You!

- Keep the underneath leg straight.
- Keep both hands on the knee.
- Keep the head facing forward.
- Elevate the hips on a folded blanket.
- In a deeper variation, the right hand is placed on the right knee.
- In the deepest variation, thread the right hand under the left thigh. Take the left hand behind the back and clasp the hands.

GOMUKHASANA: HEAD OF COW POSE

Description

- Start in Dandasana.
- Bend the left knee and bring the left foot under the right buttock.
- Bend the right knee and bring the right foot by the left hip.
- Stack the right knee directly above the left knee.
- Stretch the left arm upward by the left ear.
- Bend the left elbow, placing the hand between the shoulder blades.
- Reach the right arm behind the back and clasp the hands together (**Figure 9-12A** and **Figure 9-12B**).
- Repeat on other side.

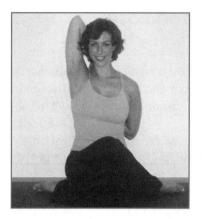
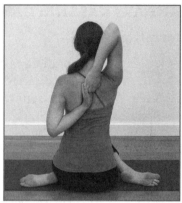

Figure 9-12A   **Figure 9-12B**

Drishti

The gaze is forward.

Alignment Cues

- Move the fleshy part of the buttocks to the sides.
- Keep both hip bones facing forward.
- Lengthen the sides of the body and draw the ribcage toward the spine.
- Point the lifted elbow toward the ceiling.
- Keep the chin parallel to the floor and drawn inward.

Benefits

This pose will:

- Increase circulation in the shoulder and knee joints
- Open the hips
- Open the chest
- Stimulate deep breathing
- Tone and strengthen the abdominal and lower back muscles

Modifications or How to Make the Pose Work for You!

- Perform the arm position of this pose in Tadasana or Easy pose.
- Use a strap behind the back to enable the hands to grasp.
- Place a blanket or two under the hips.

CHAKRAVAKASANA: CAT/DOG POSE

Description

- Start on all fours with the hands directly under the shoulders and the knees directly under the hips. Maintain a neutral spine.
- Lengthen from the tailbone to the crown of the head (**Figure 9-13A**).
- Initiating the movement from the core, round the back, drawing the tailbone under and taking the chin toward the chest (**Figure 9-13B**).
- Reverse the action by initiating the movement from the core and tilting the tailbone upward and lifting the chest and head (**Figure 9-13C**).
- Repeat several times.

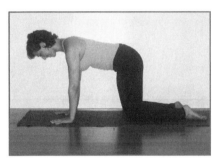

Figure 9-13A

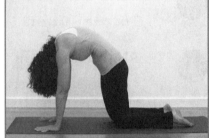

Figure 9-13B

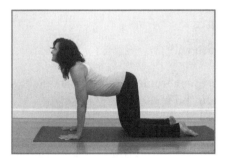

Figure 9-13C

Drishti

The gaze is toward the navel in Cat and forward in Dog.

Alignment Cues

- With the palms firmly on the ground, extend the thumbs toward each other and spread and engage the fingers.
- Draw the shoulder blades down the back.
- Keep the arms straight.
- Move slowly, sequentially, and rhythmically through the movement of this asana, feeling the movement through the vertebrae.
- In Cat, keep the head heavy and draw the navel toward the spine.
- In Dog, float the chest forward and draw the shoulder blades together.

Benefits

This pose will:

- Create spinal flexibility
- Develop abdominal strength
- Develop back strength
- Promote balance
- Promote relaxation and calm the mind

Modifications or How to Make the Pose Work for You!

- Use a blanket under the knees.
- If the wrists are sensitive, place the elbows and lower arms on the floor.
- Start on all fours and extend the right arm and the left leg. Keep the hips level and the spine in Tadasana. Repeat on the other side.

VIRASANA: HERO POSE

Description

- Kneel on the yoga mat with the knees hip-width apart and the tops of the feet against the floor.
- Lower the buttocks to the floor between the ankles.
- Rest the palms on the tops of the thighs (**Figure 9-14**).

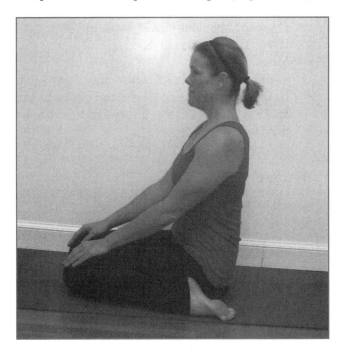

Figure 9-14

Drishti

The gaze is forward or eyes can be closed.

Alignment Cues

- Press the tops of the toes evenly against the floor.
- Lengthen the feet backward.
- Lift the hips slightly to rotate the flesh of the calves outward.
- Lift and open the chest.

- Lengthen the tailbone downward.
- Roll the shoulder blades down the back.
- Lift the crown of the head upward.

 ## Benefits

This pose will:

- Stretch the quadriceps and muscles surrounding the ankles
- Strengthen the spine and stretch the chest
- Develop a strong seated posture for meditation

 ## Modifications or How to Make the Pose Work for You!

- Place a block under the buttocks and sit on the block.
- Open a blanket so it extends from the knees to the tops of the feet.
- Place a folded blanket under the tops of the feet.
- Place a folded blanket in the crease of the knee (**Figure 9–15**).

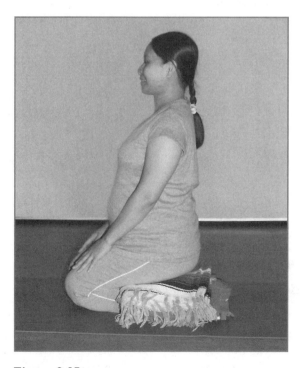

Figure 9-15

- If the tailbone touches the floor and the thighs are together, practice Supta Virasana. Place the hands by the toes and slowly lower onto one elbow at a time. Take the tailbone toward the knees. Lower one shoulder at a time to the floor. Stretch the arms overhead and hold the elbows (**Figure 9-16**). This can also be performed with a bolster under the back. This pose is excellent for pregnancy when using the bolster (**Figure 9-17**).

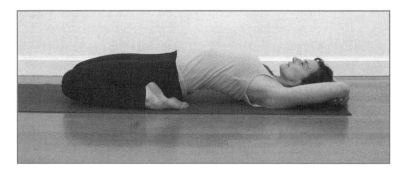

Figure 9-16

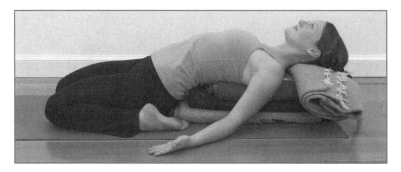

Figure 9-17

PARIGHASANA: GATE POSE

Description

- Start by kneeling with the hips and torso in Tadasana.
- Extend the right leg directly to the side with the sole of the foot on the floor.
- The toes and knee face forward.

- Slide the right arm down the right leg.
- Lift the left arm overhead, extending fully through the side of the body from the knee through the fingertips.
- Bend laterally to the right with the left arm (**Figure 9-18**).
- Repeat on the other side.

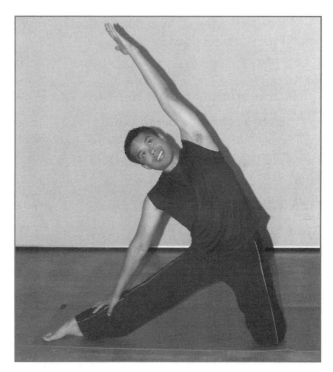

Figure 9-18

Drishti

The gaze is either toward the extended leg, directly forward, or toward the lifted arm.

Alignment Cues

- Maintain the arm overhead next to the ear.
- Draw the kneecap upward to fully engage the leg.
- Draw the ribcage inward toward the spine.
- Drop the tailbone downward.
- Keep the hip bones and ribcage directly forward.

Benefits

This pose will:

*   Deeply stretch the lateral muscles of the torso
*   Stimulate deep breathing
*   Strengthen the abdominal muscles
*   Promote flexibility in the spine
*   Develop balance

Modifications or How to Make the Pose Work for You!

*   Place a blanket under the knee.
*   Allow the baby toe side of the foot to come off the floor and extend through the sole of the foot.

KAPOTASANA: PIGEON POSE

Description

*   Start on all fours.
*   Bring the right leg forward, bending the right knee to the ground.
*   Drop the right thigh to the ground.
*   Stretch the left leg directly back, extending through the heel and toes.
*   Place the hands on the ground in a position where the chest lifts and the shoulder blades drop (**Figure 9–19A**).
*   Walk the hands as far forward as possible and release the torso and forehead to the ground (**Figure 9–19B**).
*   Repeat on the other side.

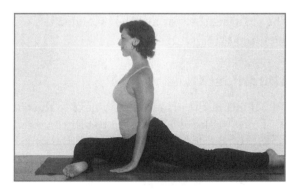

Figure 9-19A

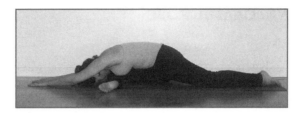

Figure 9-19B

Drishti

The gaze is forward toward the third eye or with eyes closed.

Alignment Cues

- Keep the hips and shoulders in Tadasana.
- Before lowering the torso, align the shoulders directly over the hips.
- Drop the tailbone and sacrum down.
- Balance the buttocks evenly on the floor.
- Keep the front knee in line with the front hip.
- The back leg is fully engaged.
- The back knee and top of foot face the floor.

Benefits

This pose will:

- Stretch and bring circulation to the hips, buttocks, and thighs
- Elongate the spine
- Open the chest
- Stretch the abdominal cavity

Modifications or How to Make the Pose Work for You!

- Place an appropriate height blanket underneath the hip of the bent knee to balance the sacrum.
- Relax the chest on two folded blankets.
- Draw the front heel closer to the groin.

USTRASANA: CAMEL POSE

Description

- Kneel on a blanket with the knees parallel and hip distance apart.
- The feet face directly backward and the tops of the feet are on the floor.
- Place the hands on the lower back with the fingers facing downward.
- Draw the elbows and shoulder blades together, which lifts and opens the chest.
- Contract the abdominal and gluteal muscles as the hips and thighs go forward and the back arches.
- Release the hands to the heels with the thumbs placed on the outside.
- Allow the head to drop back, keeping the back of the neck elongated (**Figure 9-20**).

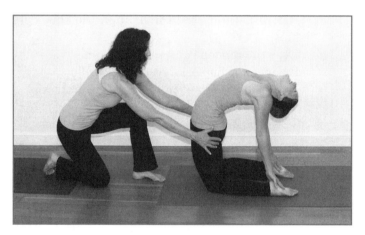

Figure 9-20

 ## Drishti

The gaze is upward.

 ## Alignment Cues

- Draw the tailbone downward toward the knees as the hip bones press forward.
- Keep the shins and feet parallel to each other.
- Keep both hip bones facing forward.

- Move the back of the heart forward and upward.
- Firmly engage the buttock muscles to protect the back.
- Lengthen the back of the neck so there is no pressure on the cervical spine.

Benefits

This pose will:

- Expand the lungs
- Increase spinal flexibility
- Stretch the quadriceps, abdominals, and pectorals
- Strengthen the buttocks, lower back, and neck muscles

Modifications or Ways to Make the Pose Work for You!

- Turn the toes under.
- Keep the hands on the lower back and work on opening the chest.
- Place the front of the body on a wall and keep the thighs in contact with the wall as the hands drop to the heels.
- Make a shawl from a blanket. Place it behind the neck. Cross both ends of the blanket in front of the sternum and hold the ends with the hands. This adds support for the neck (**Figure 9–21**).

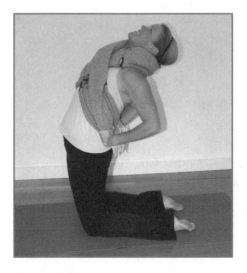

Figure 9-21

STUDY QUESTIONS

1. Describe three alignment cues for Dandasana. How does this pose create better posture?
2. What structural parts of Dandasana are inherent in Baddha Konasana?
3. In Navasana, how is balance achieved?
4. What emotional and psychological elements do you experience while practicing the backbend Ustrasana?
5. Describe three modifications for Upavistha Konasana.

 # YOGA MOMENT

Practice Paschimottanasana (Seated Forward Fold pose) using one, two, or even three blankets on your thighs to support the head. Let the forehead relax completely and evenly on the blankets. Close the eyes. Stay in this pose for five minutes. Record your observations.

CHAPTER TEN

Prone and Supine Poses

Open Your Heart

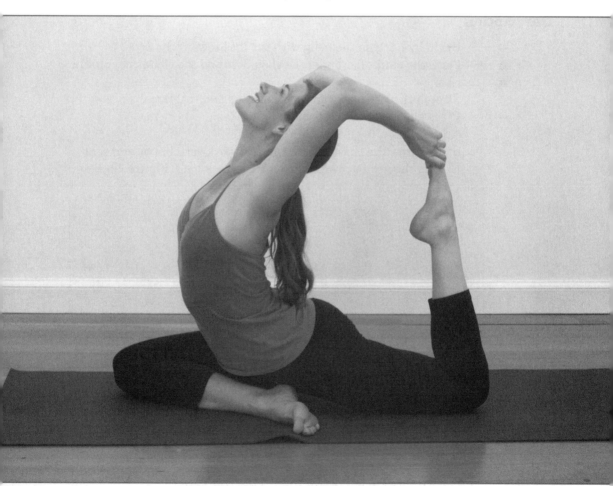

Blessed are the flexible, for they shall not be bent out of shape.

— **Anonymous**

These groups of **prone** and **supine** poses develop back strength and flexibility while creating a healthy spine.

PRONE POSES

BHUJANGASANA: COBRA POSE

Description

- Begin by lying on the belly with the face toward the floor.
- Place the palms flat under the shoulders and the elbows next to the ribs.
- Stretch the legs backward and keep the feet together.
- Press all ten toes into the floor.
- Anchor the tailbone downward.
- Slowly draw the chest forward and upward, vertebra by vertebra.
- Extend the head upward and keep the neck long (**Figure 10-1**).

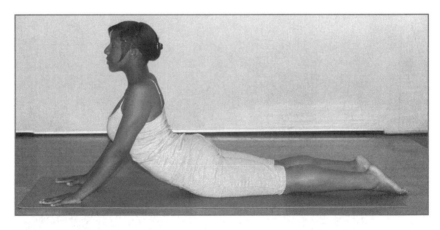

Figure 10-1

 Drishti

The gaze is forward or upward toward the third eye.

Alignment Cues

- Keep the legs and buttock muscles fully engaged.
- Keep both hip bones on the floor.
- Stretch both sides of the body equally.
- Draw the shoulder blades down the back, creating as much distance as possible between the ears and shoulders.
- Keep the elbows close to the ribs and facing backward.
- Create a balanced curve in the spine without putting pressure on the lower back.
- Lengthen the neck without constricting the cervical spine.

Benefits

This pose will:

- Create flexibility and strength in the spine
- Stimulate the thyroid and parathyroid glands
- Open the chest
- Open the heart space
- Strengthen the legs

Modifications or How to Make the Pose Work for You!

- Allow space between the feet and legs.
- Decrease the lift of the torso.
- Keep the gaze downward and the head facing forward.
- To build back strength, lift the palms slightly off the floor for five seconds while reaching the crown of the head forward.

DHANURASANA: BOW POSE

Description

- Start by lying on the belly with the hands at the side and the chin on the floor.
- Bend the knees so the lower legs are perpendicular to the floor.
- Reach the arms backward and grab the outside of the feet.
- Keep the thumb with the other fingers.

- Squeeze the shoulder blades together and lift the torso and front of the thighs off the ground.
- Lift the crown of the head upward (**Figure 10-2**).

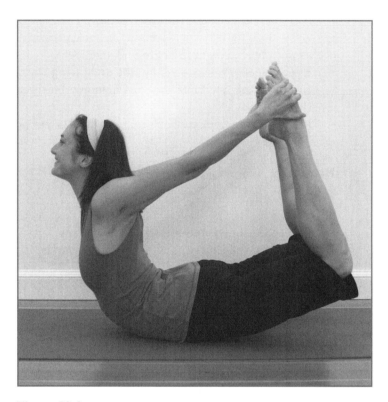

Figure 10-2

Drishti

The gaze is forward or upward toward the third eye.

Alignment Cues

- Keep the thighs parallel to each other.
- Draw the inner thighs together.
- Draw the underneath aspect of the armpits forward to open the chest.
- Create an even expansion of the spine without compressing the lower back.

- Draw the shoulders away from the ears.
- Lengthen the sides of the body.
- Keep the arms fully extended.
- Fully engage the buttock muscles.
- Press the feet firmly into the hands.

 ## Benefits

This pose will:

- Strengthen the spine
- Open the chest
- Stretch the quadriceps
- Open the heart space
- Build endurance

 ## Modifications or How to Make the Pose Work for You!

- Use a strap around the ankles (**Figure 10–3**).
- Use two blankets arranged like steps under the ribs.
- Keep the thighs on the floor.

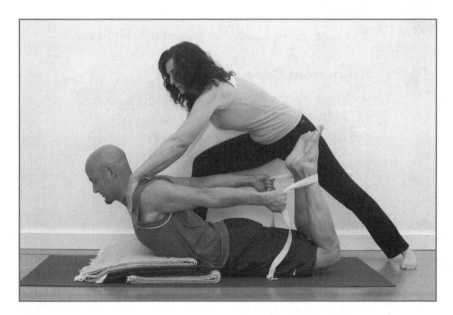

Figure 10-3

SALABHASANA: LOCUST POSE

Description

- Start on the belly with the forehead on the floor.
- Stretch the arms by the sides of the body, palms upward.
- Reach the crown of the head forward and press the tops of the feet into the floor.
- Simultaneously lift the torso and legs off the floor (**Figure 10-4**).

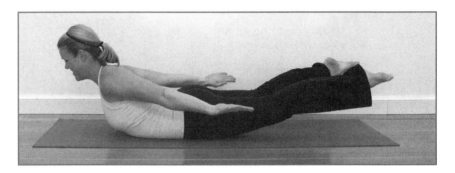

Figure 10-4

Drishti

The gaze can be forward or toward the third eye.

Alignment Cues

- Draw the shoulder blades down the back.
- Fully extend the arms and fingers.
- Energize the legs through the toes.
- Draw the tailbone toward the floor.
- Lengthen the neck.
- Open through the armpits.

Benefits

This pose will:

- Strengthen the entire spine and leg muscles
- Open the chest
- Stretch the abdominal cavity

Modifications or How to Make the Pose Work for You!

*   Only lift the legs.
*   Only lift the arms.

SUPINE POSES

SETU BANDHASANA: BRIDGE POSE

Description

*   Lie on your back with the hands at the sides of the body.
*   Bend the knees and place the soles of the feet parallel and hip distance apart.
*   Place the feet so the fingertips touch the heels.
*   Sequentially lift the buttocks and spine off the floor.
*   Roll your shoulders underneath the back until the hands clasp.
*   Draw the chin toward the chest (**Figure 10–5**).

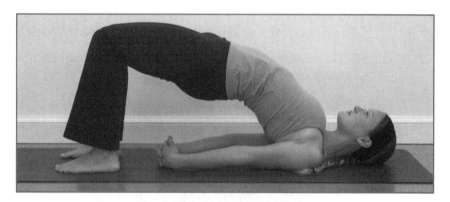

Figure 10-5

 ## Drishti

The gaze is upward or the eyes may be closed.

 ## Alignment Cues

*   Keep the thighs parallel to each other.

- Press down through the feet and extend the knees upward.
- Lengthen the thighs and pubic bone forward.
- Move the spine inward.
- Roll the biceps outward and squeeze the elbows together to open the chest.
- Lengthen the back of the neck and lift the chest toward the chin.

 ## Benefits

This pose will:

- Stretch the quadriceps
- Stretch the abdominals
- Open the chest
- Strengthen the buttocks and lower back muscles
- Promote relaxation
- Calm the mind
- Improve posture

 ## Modifications or How to Make the Pose Work for You!

- Do not clasp the hands. Keep the hands at the side of the body.
- Use a strap around the front of the ankles and grab it with the hands (**Figure 10-6**).

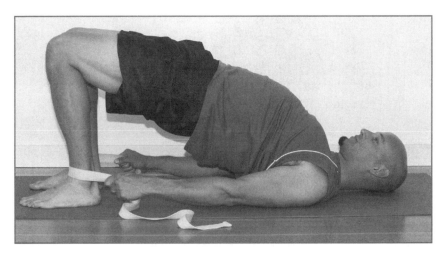

Figure 10-6

- Place a block underneath the sacrum at an appropriate height. This position is called Supported Bridge pose.

MATSYASANA: FISH POSE

Description

- Lie on the back with legs extended and feet flexed.
- Place the arms at the sides of the body.
- Bend the elbows so the palms face each other.
- Press the elbows into the floor and lift the chest, arching the back.
- Come to the top of the head, keeping the pressure on the elbows.
- Extend the arms upward and press the palms together (**Figure 10-7**).

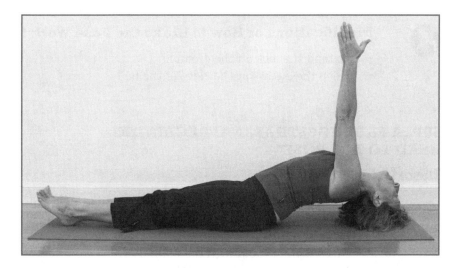

Figure 10-7

Drishti

The gaze is upward.

Alignment Cues

- Keep the elbows close to the sides of the body.
- Keep the legs fully engaged.
- Feel an imaginary string at the sternum lifting the chest to the sky.
- Do not put too much pressure on the top of the head by pressing firmly into the elbows.

Benefits

This pose will:

- Open the ribcage, chest, and abdominal cavity
- Strengthen the spine and neck muscles
- Open the heart space

Modifications or How to Make the Pose Work for You!

- Extend the legs off the ground.
- Keep the elbows at the sides of the body.

SUPTA PADANGUSTHASANA: RECLINING HEAD TO TOE POSE

Description

- Start by lying on the back in Tadasana alignment.
- Bend the right knee and hold onto the right big toe with the right index and middle fingers.
- Place the left hand with the palm down on the left thigh.
- Fully extend the left leg on the ground and flex the left foot.
- Keeping the left hip bone on the ground, extend the right leg perpendicular to the floor (**Figure 10–8**).
- Repeat on the other leg.

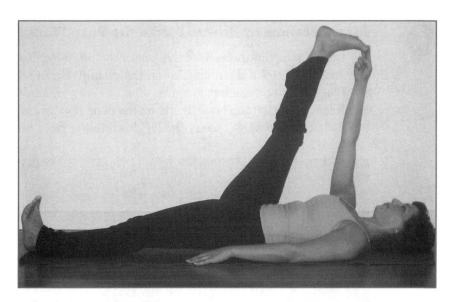

Figure 10-8

Drishti

The gaze is at the lifted big toe.

Alignment Cues

- Keep the chest and hips in Tadasana.
- Roll the shoulders back and down to open and brighten the chest.
- Create an internal rotation in both legs.
- Accentuate the energy in both legs all the way through the four corners of the feet.
- Keep the back of the neck long.

Benefits

This pose will:

- Stretch the hamstring and groin muscles
- Bring circulation into the knee
- Promote postural awareness

Modifications or How to Make the Pose Work for You!

*   Loop a strap on the arch of the foot of the lifted leg. Keep the arms straight and the shoulders flat on the ground (**Figure 10-9**).
*   Place a blanket under the neck.
*   Keeping the left hip bone firmly on the floor, revolve the right thighbone outward as you carry the leg down to the right side.

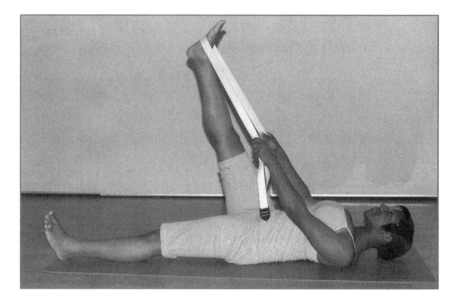

Figure 10-9

APANASANA: KNEES TO CHEST POSE

Description

*   Lie flat on the back in Tadasana alignment.
*   Draw both knees into the chest.
*   Hold the elbows below the knees (**Figure 10-10**).

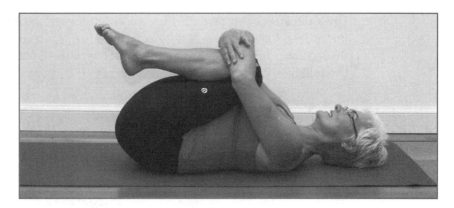

Figure 10-10

Drishti

The gaze is upward or eyes are closed.

Alignment Cues

- Draw the shoulder blades down the back.
- Keep the back of the neck long.
- Keep the chest open.
- Drop the tailbone down to lengthen the spine.

Benefits

This pose will:

- Stretch the lower back
- Relieve lower back pain
- Stimulate the digestive organs
- Calm the mind
- Promote relaxation

Modifications or How to Make the Pose Work for You!

- Place the hands on the knees.
- Place a blanket under the neck.
- Massage the lower back by rolling from side to side.

- Open the knees and grab the inside of the arches of the feet. Let the knees drop toward the ground. Keep the shins perpendicular to the floor. Allow each vertebra to be in contact with the floor and release the tailbone. This position is called Happy Baby pose.

JATHARA PARIVARTANASANA: SUPINE TWIST POSE
Description

- Start by lying on the back with legs stretched upward, perpendicular to the floor, and the arms extended to the sides with the palms facing upward.
- Bend the knees to the chest.
- Roll the knees to the left side as the gaze turns to the right (**Figure 10-11**).
- Repeat to the other side.

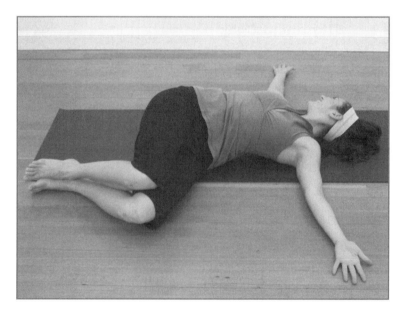

Figure 10-11

Drishti

The gaze is toward the thumb of the hand opposite the knees.

Alignment Cues

- Keep both shoulders rooted to the floor.
- Keep both sides of the body long.

Benefits

This pose will:

- Stretch the lower back and neck
- Relieve lower back pain
- Open the chest
- Promote relaxation

Modifications or How to Make the Pose Work for You!

- Bend the right knee and twist to the left. Keep the left leg straight and use the left hand on the right knee to increase the stretch. Repeat on other side (**Figure 10–12**).

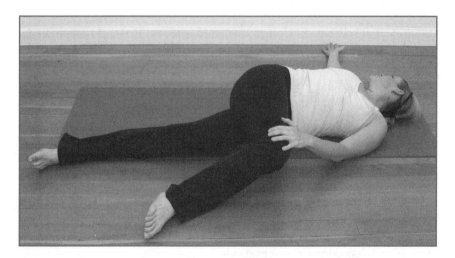

Figure 10-12

- Cross the right leg over the left, press the lower back into the floor, and drop both knees to the left. Repeat on other side (**Figure 10–13**).

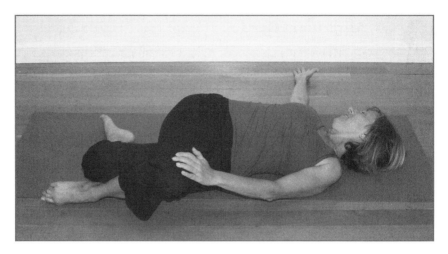

Figure 10-13

STUDY QUESTIONS

1. What do Cobra, Locust, Fish, and Bow all have in common?
2. Describe three alignment cues for Bhujangasana.
3. What are three modifications for Supta Padangusthasana?
4. What are three benefits for Setu Bandhasana?
5. What are three benefits for Apanasana?

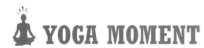 YOGA MOMENT

Practice Bridge pose three times: first, with the hands interlaced under the hips; second, with a strap wrapped around the ankles; and, third, with a block under the sacrum. Stay in each variation for five breaths. Record your observations.

CHAPTER ELEVEN

Inversions

Face Your Fears

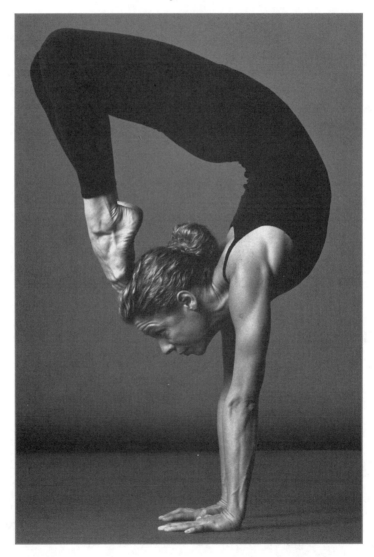

*I'm through accepting limits 'cause someone says
they're so. Some things I cannot change but 'til
I try, I'll never know. It's time to try Defying gravity.
I think I'll try defying gravity. And you can't pull
me down.*

— **From *Wicked*, music and lyrics by Stephen Schwartz**

Inversions are especially beneficial to the circulatory and digestive systems because you are moving the blood and lymph toward the heart. Inversions can also be scary. People are afraid of going upside down. The inversions we describe are a good start for overcoming fear and gaining body awareness.

Yoga Science

Yoga asanas are known to bolster the immune system, for they promote the formation of both white and red blood vessels. The inversions encourage optimal circulation of the body fluids. This speeds the delivery of disease-fighting cells to the sites of infection and helps transport infectious agents to the lymphatic tissue (Robin, 2002, pp. 390).

INVERSIONS

Plow pose and Shoulder Stand have a direct effect on the proper functioning of the thyroid and parathyroid glands, which are situated in the neck region. Due to the firm chin lock their blood supply is increased (Ivengar, 1979, pp. 213).

HALASANA: PLOW POSE

Description

- Start by lying on the back with the legs extended toward the ceiling and the arms at the sides of the body.

- Bring the legs over the head until the toes touch the floor.
- Press into the balls of the feet.
- Roll the shoulders under the back and clasp the hands together resting them on the floor.
- Draw the chin toward the chest (**Figure 11–1**).

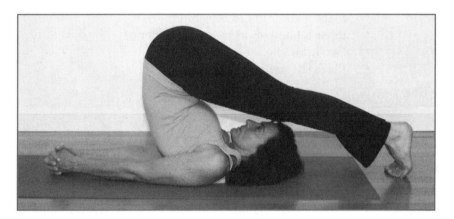

Figure 11-1

Drishti

The gaze is toward the center of the heart with eyes open or closed.

Alignment Cues

- Keep the back of the neck long with no pressure on the cervical spine.
- Do not turn the head during this pose.
- Keep the lower back rounded and the navel drawn in toward the spine.
- Fully engage the legs and spread the toes.
- Draw the elbows together and press the baby fingers into the floor.

Benefits

This pose will:

- Stretch the back, shoulders, and neck
- Promote healthy digestion and elimination

- Stimulate the thyroid gland
- Improve circulation

 Modifications or How to Make the Pose Work for You!

- Place a bolster or blankets under the feet.
- Place a chair under the shins.
- Place a blanket under the shoulders.
- Bend the knees by the ears.
- Place the palms under the toes.

SARVANGASANA: SHOULDER STAND

Description

- Lie on the back with two blankets under the shoulders.
- Draw the knees into the chest.
- Extend the legs over the head so that the buttocks and hips are off the floor and the knees are in line with the eyes.
- Place the hands on the lower back with the fingers facing the tailbone.
- Roll the elbows inward, making the upper arms parallel to each other.
- Move the hands up the back and draw the shoulders together.
- Keep the spine long, the legs active, and the toes spread (**Figure 11-2**).
- To release, slowly roll the spine to the floor using the hands for support.

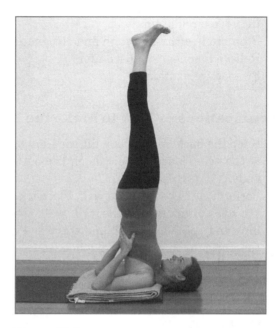

Figure 11-2

Drishti

The gaze is at the center of the heart with the eyes open or closed.

Alignment Cues

- **Do not turn the head.**
- Keep the back of the neck fully elongated.
- The shoulders, hips, and legs are in Tadasana.
- Draw the upper arms close in to the body.
- Draw the tailbone inward to fully extend the trunk and legs.
- Keep the legs perpendicular to the floor.
- Move the chest toward the chin.
- Walk the hands up the back to lengthen the spine.
- Extend through the balls of the feet.

Benefits

This pose will:

- Stretch the neck, shoulders, and upper back
- Strengthen the neck

- Improve circulation
- Promote healthy digestion and elimination
- Relieve menopausal discomfort
- Promote relaxation

Modifications or How to Make the Pose Work for You!

- Keep the back on the floor, lift the hips, and keep the knees in front of the eyes. Place the hands on the buttocks to support the lower body.
- Perform this pose using a wall. Place the hips against the wall and the soles of the feet on the wall. Walk the feet up the wall until the hips and spine are lifted and there is a straight line created from the knees to the chest. Take one leg at a time away from the wall when comfortable and stable.

STUDY QUESTIONS

1. What is the most important rule to remember when practicing Plow pose and Shoulder Stand?
2. What are two physiological benefits of inversions?
3. Describe three alignment cues for Halasana.
4. What are the benefits for Sarvangasana?
5. Describe three modifications for Halasana.

YOGA MOMENT

Practice Shoulder Stand for as long as you can comfortably and correctly maintain it. Close your eyes. Breathe in for the count of five, retain the breath for the count of five, and then exhale for the count of five. Do not strain. Record your observations.

CHAPTER 12

Restorative Poses

Regroup and Renew!

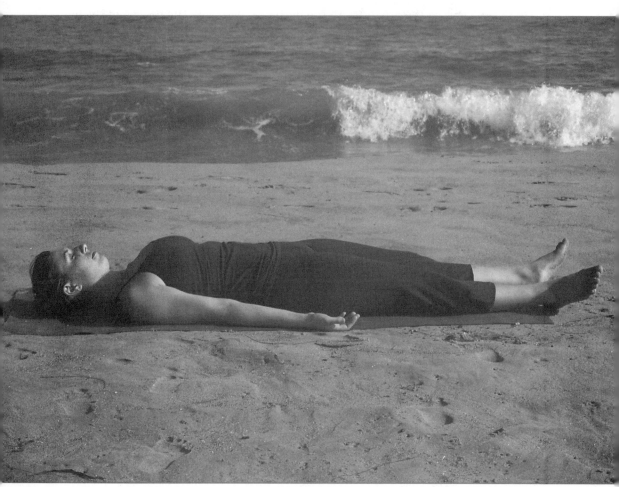

Stop the words now. Open the window on the door of your heart. And let the spirits fly in and out.

— **Rumi**

RESTORATIVE POSES
BALASANA: CHILD'S POSE
Description

- Sit on the ground with the buttocks resting on the heels and the big toes touching.
- Keep the shoulders over the hips and the palms resting on the thighs.
- Keeping the big toes touching, separate the knees and lower the chest to the thighs and forehead to the floor.
- Release the arms to the floor next to the torso with the palms facing upward (**Figure 12-1**).

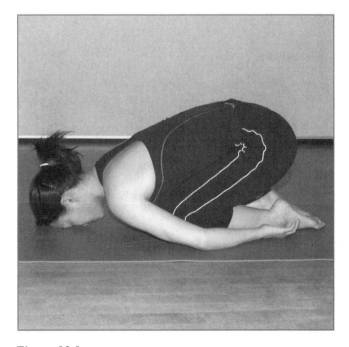

Figure 12-1

Drishti

The gaze is to the ground or eyes are closed.

Alignment Cues

- The buttocks rest completely on the heels.
- Drop the tailbone toward the heels.
- Take the shoulder blades down the back.
- Let the upper arms drape down toward the floor.
- Allow the forehead to rest fully and perfectly balanced on the floor.
- Soften the abdominal muscles.

Benefits

This pose will:

- Stretch and lengthen the back
- Stretch the ankles and shins
- Calm and quiet the mind
- Release lower back and shoulder tension
- Relax the neck and facial muscles

Modifications or How to Make the Pose Work for You!

- Fully extend the arms overhead so that the elbows lift off the floor. Energize the fingers and spread them wide (**Figure 12-2**).
- Use a blanket under the buttocks if the buttocks do not touch the heels.
- Use a blanket under the forehead if more support is needed.
- For a more restful variation, use a bolster under the abdomen.

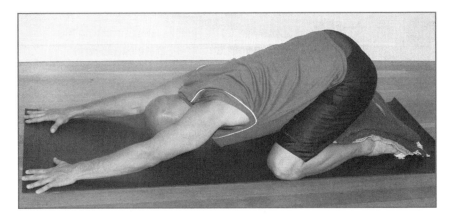

Figure 12-2

VIPARITA KARANI: LEGS UP THE WALL POSE

Description

- Place a bolster or two folded blankets against the wall.
- Sit on the bolster or blankets with the right hip against the wall.
- Revolve the hips toward the wall and then lift the legs up the wall.
- Using hands for support, lower the back to the floor.
- Place the arms at the sides of the body with the palms upward, or bend the elbows even with the shoulders, moving the upper arms toward the ears and the palms up (**Figure 12-3**).
- Close the eyes.

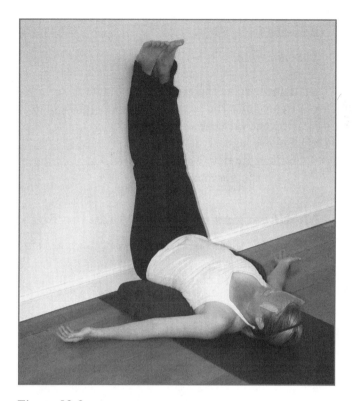

Figure 12-3

Drishti

Close the eyes and bring the gaze and the awareness inward.

Alignment Cues

- Perfectly balance the right and left sides of the body.
- Drop the shoulders away from the ears.
- Soften all the muscles of the face.
- Relax the jaw and brow.
- Release the lower back to the support.
- Completely let go!

Benefits

This pose will:

- Totally relax the body
- Rejuvenate the circulation and regulate blood pressure
- Prevent varicose veins and edema
- Relieve leg fatigue
- Relieve anxiety
- Calm the nervous system

Modifications or How to Make the Pose Work for You!

- Practice the pose without a bolster or blanket. This is very soothing for the back.
- Practice with the hips on the floor and the bolster resting on the abdomen.
- Place a blanket under the head for extra support.
- Use an eye pillow over the eyes.
- For stretching the inner thighs, straddle the legs or place the soles of the feet together and allow the knees to open.

SUPTA BADDHA KONASANA: SUPPORTED BOUND ANGLE POSE

Description

- Sit in Dandasana with a bolster behind the buttocks and a folded blanket on the end of the bolster to support the neck.
- Bring the soles of the feet together and allow the knees to move apart from each other.
- Make a loop with the strap so that the loose end is by the dominant hand and is facing backward.
- Put the belt over the head and loop it around the baby toe side of the feet. Position the belt by the sacrum.
- Place the hands evenly on the floor by the hips and extend the spine upward.
- Slowly release the back to the bolster.
- Tighten the strap so that the heels move closer to the groin.

- Relax the arms at the side with the palms facing upward (**Figure 12-4**).
- Close the eyes.

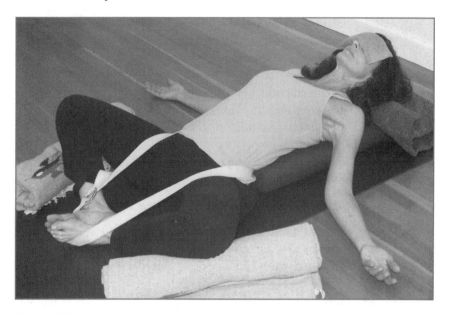

Figure 12-4

Drishti

Close the eyes and bring the gaze and awareness inward.

Alignment Cues

- Make sure the strap is placed at the sacrum and not at the waist.
- Create a downward slope from the forehead to the chin using blankets if necessary.
- Find perfect balance in the body from right to left.
- Draw the shoulders down the back.
- Widen the groin.
- Relax the elbows to the floor.
- Allow the fingers to soften and naturally curl.
- Soften all the muscles and bones of the face.

Benefits

This pose will:

- Stretch and open the thighs, knees, and groin
- Lift the chest, which enhances respiration
- Relax the abdominal organs
- Reduce fatigue
- Relieve headaches
- Lessen menstrual and menopausal symptoms
- Promote balance in reproductive organs in both males and females
- Calm the mind and promote relaxation

Modifications or How to Make the Pose Work for You!

- Place rolled blankets under the thighs for additional support.
- Do not use the strap. Use the rolled blankets.
- Cross the legs in Easy pose. After a few minutes, switch the cross of the legs.
- Use an eye pillow.

Yoga Science

During Savasana, the parasympathetic nervous system becomes dominant. The slow, rhythmic breathing decreases the signals to the hypothalamus, a region of the brain that functions as the main control center. This resets the blood pressure to a lower level.

In a study focusing on Savasana as a treatment for hypertension (high blood pressure), scientists found—on average—that the mean blood pressure dropped significantly with the daily practice of thirty minutes of Savasana over a period of several months. For subjects already taking medication for high blood pressure, the practice of Savasana led to a reduction in the use of medication by 32% (Robin, 2002, pp. 338).

SAVASANA: CORPSE POSE

Description

- Lie flat on the back.
- Place the arms about eight inches from the sides of the body with the palms facing upward.
- Let the thighs roll outward (**Figure 12–5**).
- Close the eyes.

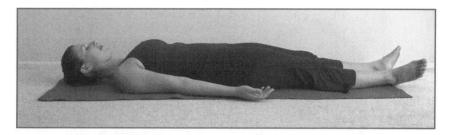

Figure 12-5

Drishti

Take the gaze and awareness inward.

Alignment Cues

- Roll the shoulders and biceps outward.
- Allow the feet to roll outward.
- Draw the tailbone downward toward the feet.
- Soften the hands and allow the fingers to naturally curl.
- Relax every muscle in the body.
- Release the bones.
- Soften everywhere!

Benefits

This pose will:

- Assimilate and integrate all the benefits of the yoga practice
- Reduce stress
- Relieve anxiety

- Calm the nervous system
- Rejuvenate the body's energy
- Allow you to experience peace and joy

Modifications or How to Make the Pose Work for You!

- Use an eye pillow.
- Place a bolster or one or two rolled blankets under the knees.
- Elevate the calves and heels with one or two folded blankets.
- Place a folded blanket or bolster under the back (this is called Supported Savasana).
- Place a folded blanket under the back of the head to keep the back of the neck long.

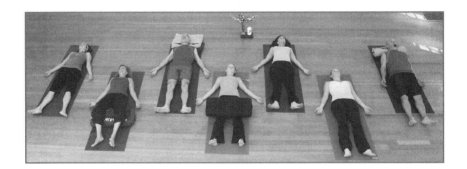

STUDY QUESTIONS

1. What are three benefits of practicing restorative poses?
2. How do restorative poses affect the nervous system?
3. Describe three alignment cues for Supta Baddha Konasana.
4. Describe three modifications for Viparita Karani.
5. Why is Savasana practiced at the end of a yoga session?

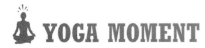

YOGA MOMENT

At the end of your day, at your home, practice Viparita Karani for five minutes. Close your eyes. Go inward. Record your observations.

CHAPTER THIRTEEN

Sun Salutations

Energize Your Life

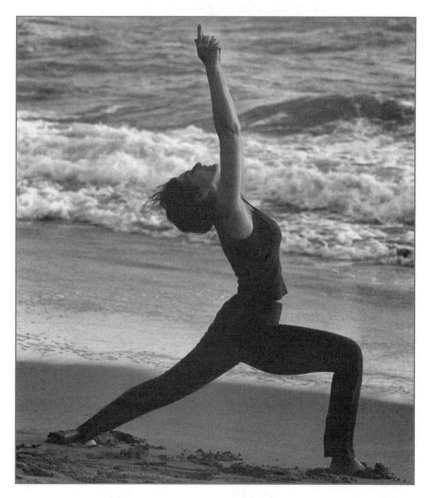

Far away, there in the sunshine, are my highest aspirations. I may not reach them, but I can look up and see their beauty, believe in them, and try to follow where they lead.

— **Louisa May Alcott**

Sun Salutations, in Sanskrit called Surya Namaskar, involve integrating breath with movement to create a flowing sequence of asanas that heat the body. These synchronized movements that increase awareness of breath and body are traditionally practiced before sunrise. They are usually incorporated into a class as a way to create heat for the practice while warming the muscles and joints. Other benefits include developing strength, flexibility, grace, stamina, focus, and coordination. Many variations of Sun Salutations exist. Three commonly practiced variations are described here.

SURYA NAMASKAR A: SUN SALUTATION A

1. Begin in Mountain pose with feet together or hip-width apart. Hands are in Prayer pose (**Figure 13-1**).
2. Inhale. Sweep the arms overhead and gaze upward (**Figure 13-2**).

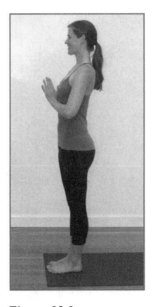 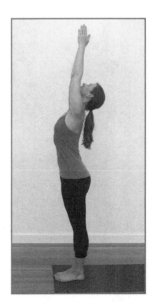

Figure 13-1   Figure 13-2

3. Exhale. Forward Fold. Bring the forehead to the knees (**Figure 13-3**).
4. Inhale. Forward Bend. Create a flat back (**Figure 13-4**).

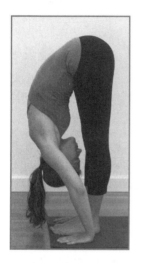 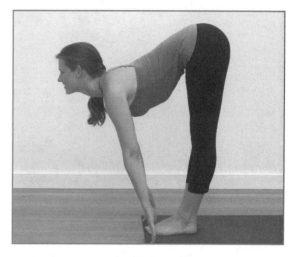

Figure 13-3   **Figure 13-4**

5. Exhale. Step or jump into Plank pose, and then lower the body to the floor (**Figure 13-5A** and **Figure 13-5B**).

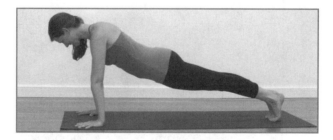

Figure 13-5A

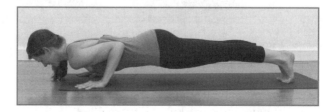

Figure 13-5B

6. Inhale. Lift to Cobra or Upward Facing Dog (**Figure 13-6**).

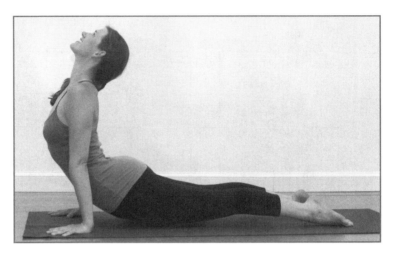

Figure 13-6

7. Exhale. Release Cobra and push into Downward Facing Dog. Take five deep Ujjayi breaths (**Figure 13-7**).

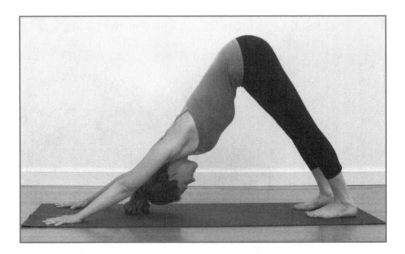

Figure 13-7

8. Inhale. Lift head. Look between hands. Jump or step forward to Forward Bend. Back is flat (**Figure 13-8**).
9. Exhale. Forward Fold (**Figure 13-9**).

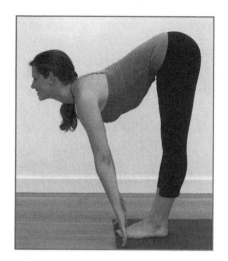

Figure 13-8

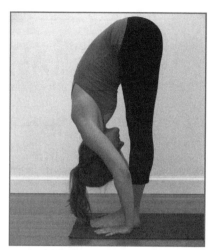

Figure 13-9

10. Inhale. Sweep arms overhead (**Figure 13–10**).
11. Exhale. Mountain pose with hands in Prayer pose (**Figure 13–11**).

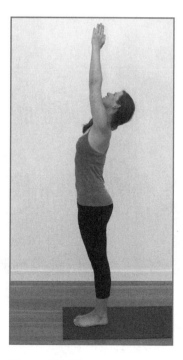

Figure 13-10

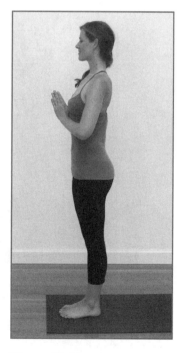

Figure 13-11

Student Testimonial

"As an athlete I move in quick, explosive bursts. The Sun Saluta-tions complement my activities by moving my body in a rhythmic and flowing manner."

SURYA NAMASKAR B: SUN SALUTATION B

1. Start in Mountain pose with the hands in Prayer position (**Figure 13-12**).
2. Inhale. Sweep the arms overhead and bend the knees into Chair pose (**Figure 13-13**).

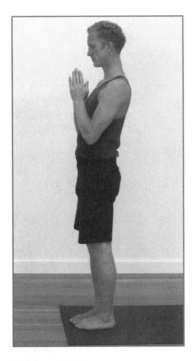
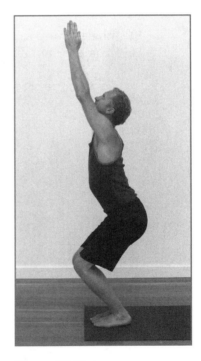

Figure 13-12   Figure 13-13

3. Exhale. Forward Fold. Bring the forehead to the knees (**Figure 13-14**).
4. Inhale. Forward Bend. Create a flat back (**Figure 13-15**).

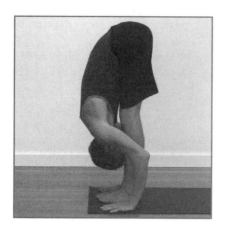 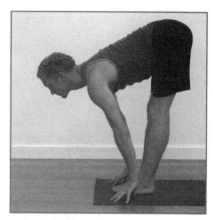

Figure 13-14   **Figure 13-15**

5. Exhale. Step or jump into Plank pose, and then lower the body to the floor (**Figure 13-16A** and **Figure 13-16B**).

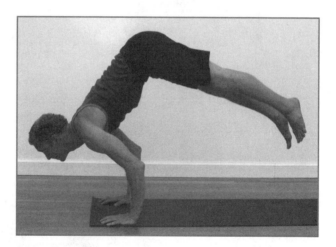

Figure 13-16A

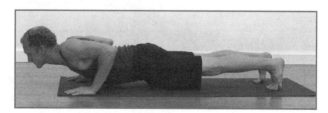

Figure 13-16B

6. Inhale. Lift to Cobra or Upward Facing Dog (**Figure 13–17**).

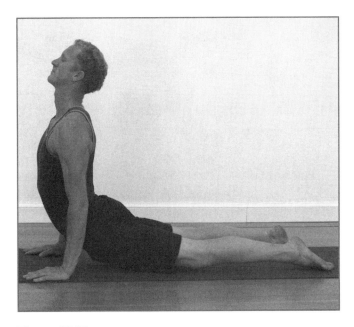

Figure 13-17

7. Exhale. Push back to Downward Facing Dog (**Figure 13–18**).

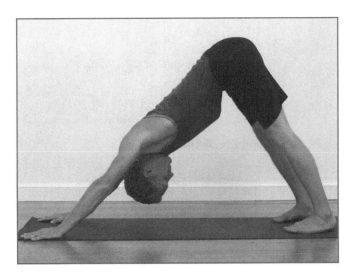

Figure 13-18

8. Inhale. Raise the right leg and step into Warrior I (**Figure 13-19**).

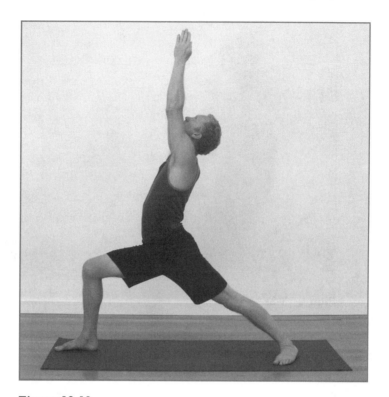

Figure 13-19

9. Exhale. Release the arms and step or jump into Plank pose. Lower the body to the floor (**Figure 13-20**).

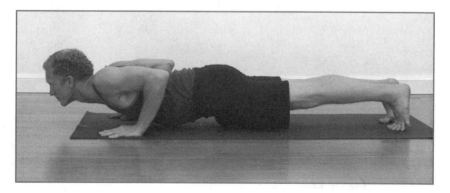

Figure 13-20

10. Inhale. Lift to Cobra or Upward Facing Dog (**Figure 13-21**).

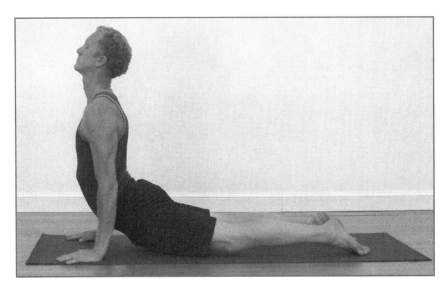

Figure 13-21

11. Exhale. Push back into Downward Facing Dog (**Figure 13-22**).

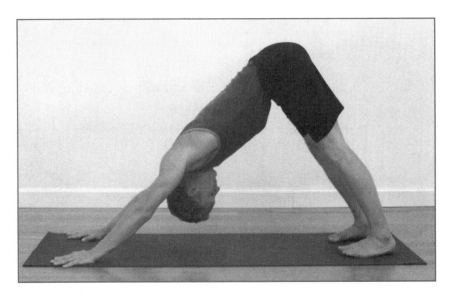

Figure 13-22

12. Inhale. Raise the left leg and step into Warrior I (**Figure 13-23**).

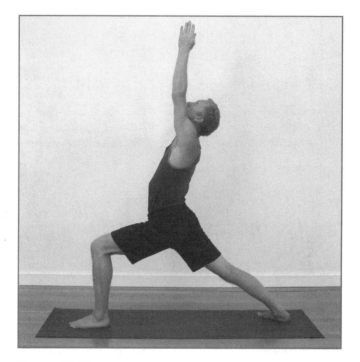

Figure 13-23

13. Exhale. Lower the arms and step or jump into Plank pose. Lower to the floor (**Figure 13-24**).

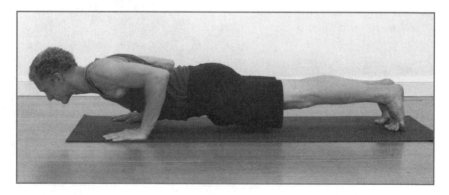

Figure 13-24

14. Inhale. Lift to Cobra or Upward Facing Dog (**Figure 13-25**).

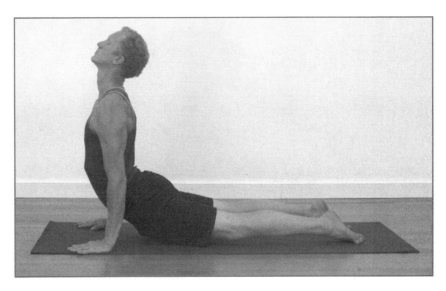

Figure 13-25

15. Exhale. Push into Downward Facing Dog. Take five breaths (**Figure 13-26**).

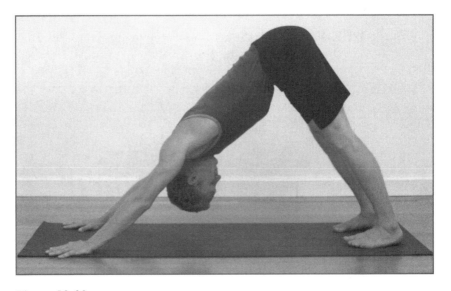

Figure 13-26

16. Inhale. Bend the knees, look between the hands, and step or jump feet together to Forward Bend (**Figure 13-27A**). Create a flat back (**Figure 13-27B**).

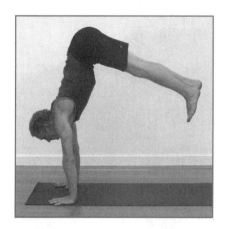

Figure 13-27A

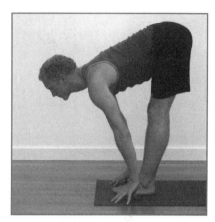

Figure 13-27B

17. Exhale. Forward Fold (**Figure 13-28**).
18. Inhale. Sweep arms to Chair pose (**Figure 13-29**).

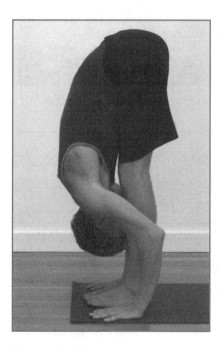
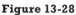

Figure 13-28

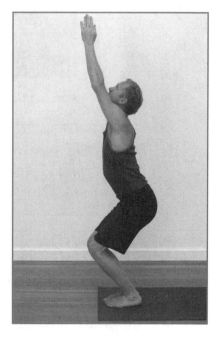

Figure 13-29

19. Exhale. Straighten the legs to Mountain pose and bring the hands to Prayer position (**Figure 13-30**).

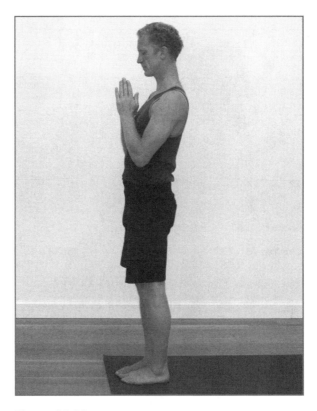

Figure 13-30

Student Testimonial

"Executing Sun Salutations allows me to enjoy full, sustained movement without ever losing sight of the breath."

SURYA NAMASKAR: CLASSICAL SUN SALUTATION WITH LUNGE

1. Stand in Mountain pose (**Figure 13-31**).
2. Inhale. Sweep the arms overhead (**Figure 13-32**).

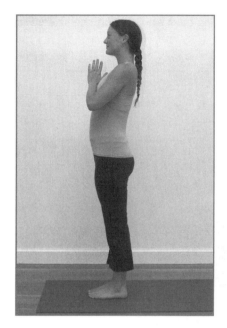

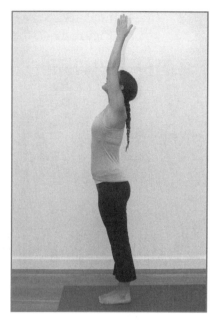

Figure 13-31   **Figure 13-32**

3. Exhale. Forward Fold. Bring the forehead to the knees. (**Figure 13-33**).
4. Inhale. Forward Bend. Create a flat back (**Figure 13-34**).

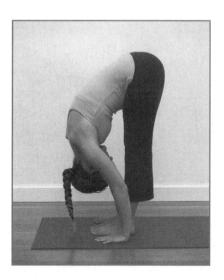

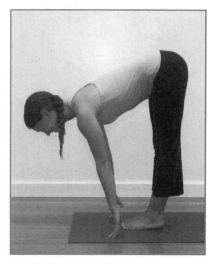

Figure 13-33   **Figure 13-34**

5. Inhale. Step the right leg back and rest on the knee. Lunge position (**Figure 13–35**).

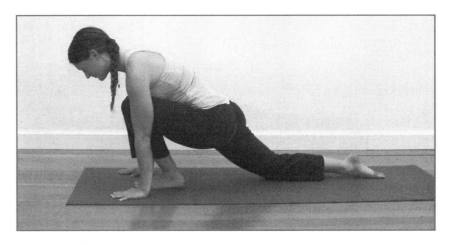

Figure 13-35

6. Exhale. Step the left foot back into Plank pose (**Figure 13–36**).

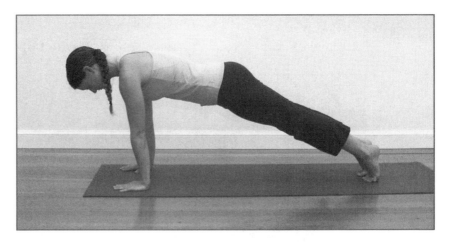

Figure 13-36

7. Continuing to exhale, lower down.
8. Inhale. Lift to Cobra or Upward Facing Dog (**Figure 13-37**).

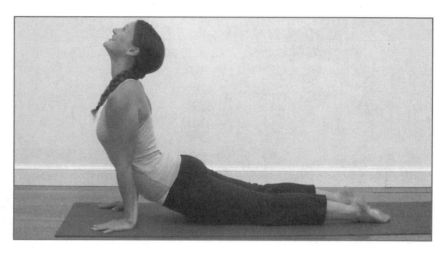

Figure 13-37

9. Exhale. Push into Downward Facing Dog (**Figure 13-38**).

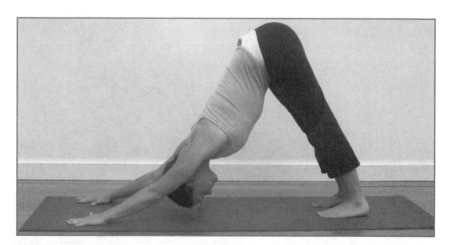

Figure 13-38

10. Inhale. Step the right foot forward. Lunge with the left knee on the ground (**Figure 13–39**).

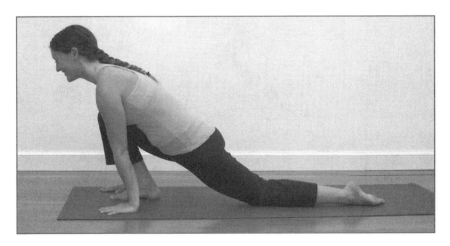

Figure 13-39

11. Exhale. Step the left foot forward to Forward Fold (**Figure 13–40**).

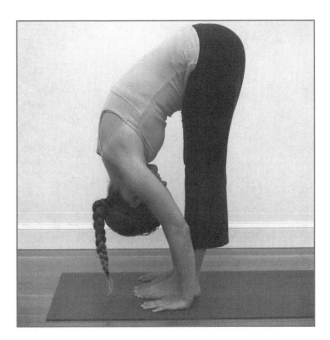

Figure 13-40

12. Inhale the arms up overhead (**Figure 13–41**).
13. Exhale. Mountain pose with hands in prayer pose (**Figure 13–42**).

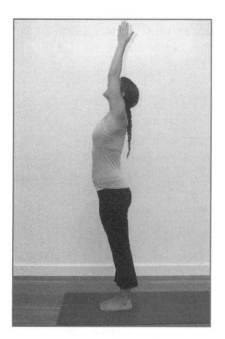

Figure 13-41

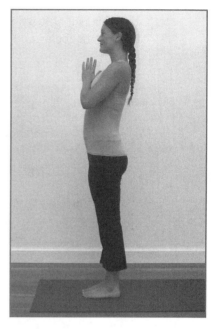

Figure 13-42

Teachers often offer modifications for each flowing series of Sun Salutations. Listen to your body's needs. Make the following modifications if necessary:

- Place the knees on the floor for Plank pose.
- Bend the knees in Forward Fold.
- Keep the hands on the thighs for Forward Bend.
- Keep the hands on the hips for Warrior I.

STUDY QUESTIONS

1. What is the purpose of Sun Salutations?
2. How can you modify the Sun Salutations?
3. Write your own testimonial for the value of Sun Salutations.
4. Describe benefits achieved with the practice of Sun Salutations.

🧘 YOGA MOMENT

Practice Sun Salutation A three times. Without judgment, be aware of the breath, the focus, and the flow of movement. Record your observations.

CHAPTER FOURTEEN

Yoga History and Philosophy

Realize Your Oneness

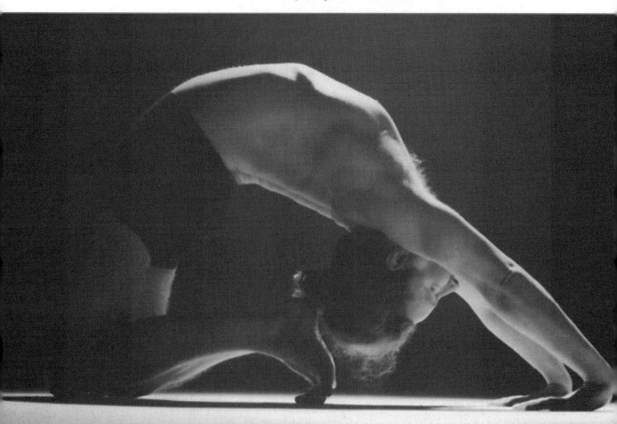

Yoga to me is an evolutionary and indeed evolving science . . . .

— **Sting**

Great debate surrounds yoga's origin, history, and practice. The yoga scriptures and teachings are so immense and complex that one could interpret its history in a myriad of ways. The swami Venkates suggested that we use ancient writings to stimulate our inquiry and to catalyze our direct perception and understanding of our own lives (White, 2007, pp. 5–6).

The purpose of this chapter is to offer a concise synopsis of yoga's history and to demonstrate how its traditions have influenced the practice as we know it today. Also described in this chapter are the major branches of yoga, the eight limbs of yoga, and the many styles of yoga.

Yoga—an ancient path to spiritual growth—is said to have originated in India over 5,000 years ago. Even though it has its roots in Hinduism, our contemporary Western approach to yoga has very little to do with any particular belief or religion (Robin, 2002). By studying yoga's roots, an appreciation of this ancient science is enhanced.

"Yoga is not a religion; it is a discipline without dogma, therefore a person of any faith or fellowship can be considered a yogi."

— **Anonymous**

It is hypothesized that ascetics living primarily in the southern portion of India developed yoga. They were vegetarians who adhered to a nonviolent philosophy, lived simply, and observed nature. These observations of animals, birds, and their own actions led to the creation of the postures we practice today. Initially, the goal of the postures was to allow these ascetics to sit still for long periods of time in meditation.

BRANCHES OF YOGA

The term *yoga* is derived from the Sanskrit word *yuj*. It is defined as "to yoke" or "to unite." Uniting the mind, the body, and the spirit is the heart of yoga philosophy. In the West, the word *yoga* is synonymous with Hatha

Yoga or the physical aspect of yoga. In India, however, throughout the centuries yoga encompassed more than just the physical aspect. There are five main branches of yoga that offer spiritual philosophies and disciplines beyond Hatha Yoga (Feuerstein, 2001). Each branch possesses unique characteristics and a particular approach to life. However, the branches can overlap, and study in one branch may stimulate involvement or study in another branch. It is important, however, to realize that modern interpretations of the branches of yoga are actually amalgams taken from many ancient and contemporary beliefs and practices (White, 2007, pp. 15).

Bhakti yoga is the yoga of devotion and selfless love (Feuerstein, 2001, pp. 36–41). Bhakti is derived from the Sanskrit word *bhaj*, which means "to serve," "to share," or "to participate." Expressing love for the Divine is demonstrated through prayer, chanting, singing, and dancing. The path of Bhakti cultivates compassion and acceptance of others. Mother Teresa and Mahatma Gandhi are two modern examples of what a Bhakti yogi represents.

Jnana yoga is the path of wisdom and is practiced by aspiring sages or scholars (Feuerstein, 2001, pp. 31–33). In Sanskrit, the word *jnana* means "knowledge" or "wisdom." These seekers study the scriptures and texts of the yoga tradition to reach enlightenment. Socrates, Kabala scholars, Jesuit priests, and Benedictine monks could all be regarded as Jnana yogis.

Karma yoga is the path of service through selfless actions without expecting anything in return (Feuerstein, 2001, pp. 47–51). Transcendence is achieved by service performed with honesty and integrity. Karma yogis help those less fortunate. The Peace Corps and Habitat for Humanity are two organizations that characterize the ideals of Karma yogis.

Raja yoga is known as the "royal" path and refers to the journey toward personal enlightenment through meditation (Feuerstein, 2001, pp. 28–29). Raja yoga's foundation integrates the "eight limbs" of yoga as outlined by Patanjali in the *The Yoga Sutras*. Examples of Raja yogis may be members of religious and spiritual communities or may pursue this path on their own.

Tantra yoga was a path of yoga accessible to all men and all women, not just the royal caste or renunciates. *Tantra* comes from two Sanskrit words: *tan* meaning "tool" and *tra* meaning "expansion." Therefore, Tantra is interpreted as "tool for expansion" or "that by which knowledge is extended or spread out" (Feuerstein, 2001, pp. 342–343). Tantra yogis do not renounce material possessions or pleasure. Tantra yogis view themselves as part of life in all its glory. They achieve self-realization through personal experimentation and experience (Isaacs, 2006). Examples of Tantra yogis may be people who live with unconditional love, acceptance, and a joy of life. Some scholars believe that **Hatha** Yoga, as we know it today, stems from Tantra yoga.

Let your life include aspects of each of the five branches of yoga: devotion, service, knowledge, contemplation, and expansion.

EIGHT LIMBS OF YOGA

Approximately 2,000 years ago the Indian sage Patanjali wrote his ancient text, *The Yoga Sutras*. These writings describe how the yoga student achieves spirituality by progressing through the eight limbs of yoga. Although Patanjali proposed that these eight limbs be explored sequentially, modern-day thinking sees the limbs like branches on a tree that can be experienced in any order. All eight "limbs" or aspects must be observed and practiced in order "to yoke" or to unify the mind, body, and soul. The eight limbs of yoga are described below in English and in Sanskrit (Iyengar, 1966).

1. *Discipline* (yama): This limb contains five moral codes to be followed: nonviolence, truthfulness, nonstealing, chastity, and greedlessness.
2. *Self-study and purification* (niyama): This limb is also divided into five codes of living: purity, contentment, austerity, study, and devotion.
3. *Posture* (asana): The first two limbs, *yama* and *niyama*, prepare the student for the practice of the third limb, *asana*. Initially, *asana* referred to the basic sitting posture. The evolution of yoga expanded the practice of *asana* to include the variety of poses we practice today. These poses are designed to stimulate every muscle, nerve, organ, gland, and energy channel in the body. By practicing asanas, the student achieves the necessary stamina, strength, and steadiness of mind to proceed to the next limbs of yoga.
4. *Breath control* (pranayama): *Pranayama* means "life force" or breath plus energy. Breath control, one of the pillars of the yoga practice, evolved as a means of controlling the mind.

5. *Sense control* (pratyahara): Practicing asanas and *pranayama* enables the student to gain control of the inner environment of the mind and senses. This allows thoughts to flow through consciousness without attachment.
6. *Concentration* (dharana): Building on the first five limbs, now the student is able to concentrate and maintain the mind in an undisturbed state. Sensations, sounds, and thoughts will not distract the student from a one-pointed focus.
7. *Meditation* (dhyana): Through deep concentration, the student arrives in a meditative state, accompanied by a peaceful, calm emotional disposition. The mind becomes empty yet keenly alert.
8. *Contemplation* (samadhi): *Samadhi* means "to bring together" or "to merge." Samadhi is the culmination and integration of the practice of all eight limbs. The student has achieved enlightenment, ecstasy, and blissful consciousness.

The practice and assimilation of the eight limbs propel the journey of the yoga student. Understanding of one limb brings insights to another.

HATHA YOGA

The physical practice of yoga is called Hatha Yoga. In his book, *Yoga Beyond Belief,* Ganga White (2007) states that "the syllable *ha* in *Hatha* means sun, which implies masculine energy and symbolizes heating, expansion, and strength; *tha* means moon, which refers to feminine energy and symbolizes cooling, contraction and flexibility. It is vitally important to bring these principles into balance."

- Hatha Yoga synthesizes limbs three and four of the eightfold path: asana (posture) and *pranayama* (breath). These two limbs create the core of Hatha Yoga.
- Hatha Yoga also means "the union of opposites."
- The science of Hatha Yoga balances and harmonizes the body's opposing energies, such as the right and left sides of the brain, the feminine and masculine aspects of the personality, and the expansion and contraction of the muscles.

- This union of opposites brings strength, vitality, and flexibility to the body, mind, and spirit.

Styles of Hatha Yoga

Under the umbrella of Hatha Yoga, many different styles exist (Kappmeier and Ambrosini, 2006). Here are some of the major styles of Hatha Yoga:

- **Iyengar yoga:** B. K. S. Iyengar developed this style. It focuses on precise physical alignment with strict attention to the detail of body positioning. This attention to detail creates a slow pace to a class. Breathing techniques are not stressed until a certain level of proficiency of the postures is attained. Props are emphasized and used to enable all levels of students to go deeper and stay longer in the poses. Music is excluded because it is thought to be a distraction.
- **Ashtanga yoga:** This vigorous style, considered the most physically demanding of all Hatha Yoga, was introduced by K. Pattabhi Jois. It is composed of six specific sequences that move from one posture to the next in an exact order. Sun Salutations, with asana variations in between, create a continuous flow of movement in these sequences. The purpose of this continuous flow is to create heat, which cleanses and detoxifies the body. Power yoga has its roots in ashtanga yoga but does not follow an exact sequence.
- **Vinyasa yoga:** This style is also referred to as "flow yoga." Sun Salutations and standing poses are linked together with the breath. Unlike ashtanga yoga, in vinyasa yoga the teacher creatively sequences the flow of the class. The word *vinyasa* means "the wind" and refers to this linking together of poses.
- **Bikram yoga:** Also known as "hot yoga," it is taught in a room kept at approximately 106 degrees Fahrenheit! Developed by Bikram Choudhury, this style has only one sequence, composed of 26 postures, executed in every class. This practice is said to detoxify the body and has also been called "yoga boot camp."
- **Kundalini yoga:** In 1969 Yogi Bhajan introduced Kundalini yoga to the Western world. This ancient practice is designed to awaken the Kundalini, or coiled energy stored at the base of the spine. The movements are fast and repetitive, with focus on rapid deep breathing or "breath of fire" and chanting. This style of yoga resembles a calisthenic workout.

- **Anasura yoga:** This style of yoga was founded in 1997 by John Friend. It blends a life-affirming Tantric yoga philosophy with emphasis on proper body alignment and community. In this spiritually uplifting style of Hatha Yoga, students are guided to fully live every moment from the heart and to see their own unique beauty and divine goodness.
- **Eclectic yoga:** This describes a blended style of yoga that does not follow one strict method or consistent routine of postures. Each teacher combines elements from many different styles, influencing the class with his or her knowledge, goals, and personality.

 Student Testimonial

"As an engineering student, I find it fascinating to experience the diverse approaches and varied scientific information presented by different yoga teachers."

YOGA TIMELINE

3000 B.C.	Archaeological findings from the Indus Valley in India reveal portraits of human beings and gods possibly practicing yoga postures (Lidell, 1993, pp. 13).
2600–1900 B.C.	Yoga artifacts found in the ancient Indian civilization called the Harappan civilization. This culture possessed high levels of technology and art. The word *yoga* appeared in their writings (Feuerstein, 2001, pp. 63, 96, 99).
2500–1000 B.C.	*The Vedas*, the oldest written record of Indian culture and yogic activities, compiles hymns and rituals praising a divine power. Vedic yoga unites the visible material world with the invisible spiritual world by sacrificing certain worldly possessions. To practice these long rituals, it was necessary to focus the mind. This inner focus became the root of yoga (Feuerstein, 2001, pp. 101–102).
800–500 B.C.	During this period, the *Upanishads*, a collection of sacred texts, reveal metaphysical speculation about

humans' place in the universe. Some of the 200 scriptures of the *Upanishads* directly relate to yoga and are about the complete connectedness of all things. Yoga is referred to as a path by which the student achieves liberation from suffering. Two yoga disciplines gained popularity at this time, karma yoga, the path of action or ritual, and jnana yoga, the path of knowledge or intense study of the scriptures. In the *Upanishads*, karma yoga demanded an internal sacrifice of the ego to achieve liberation from suffering. The intent was to be released from the cycle of cause and effect. This pursuit turned the practitioner's attention to the qualities of the inner mind. This idea was a major philosophical turning point in the evolution of yoga (Feuerstein, 2001, pp. 124–128, 134–136).

300–200 B.C.   In the *Maitrayaniya Upanishads*, another spiritual text, yoga is defined as a means of controlling the breath and the mind using the sound *OM*. This scripture describes yoga as the oneness of breath and mind, giving students an actual method or discipline for joining the universal energy with the infinite energy within. This scripture also prescribed the Six-Fold Yoga path, the precursor to Patanjali's Eight-Limbed Path (Feuerstein, 2001, pp. 206).

300 B.C.   The *Bhagavad-Gita*, described in an epic Hindu tale, provides one of the most comprehensive descriptions of yoga. The Lord Krishna instructs his pupil, Arjuna, on the ways of the world (**Figure 14-1**). The *Gita* proposed a simple approach to enlightenment consisting of karma yoga, jnana yoga, and bhakti yoga. The *Gita*, assimilated into Indian culture, remains popular today (Feuerstein, 2001, p. 187–189).

100 B.C.   A new philosophical school of metaphysical thought, called Samkhya, evolves. This school of thought reveals that every individual consists of two parts, matter (**Prakriti**) and soul (**Purusha**). The goal of yoga is to free the soul from the material world. Yoga borrows this dual cosmological system from the Samkhya tradition

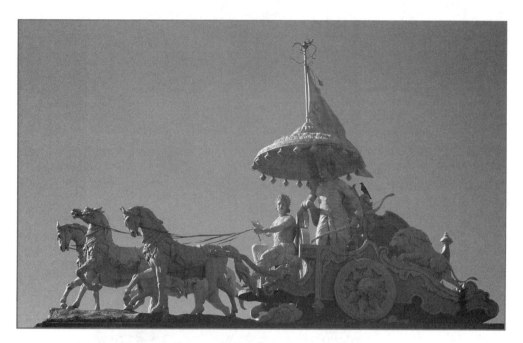

Figure 14-1 Krishna and Arjuna

and believes that the Prakriti dynamically creates everything material and Purusha passively illuminates it. Later, schools of yoga renounce all attachment to Prakriti if Purusha is to be experienced (Feuerstein, 2001, pp. 75–77).

150–200 A.D. Patanjali (**Figure 14-2**), *the father of modern yoga*, authored a collection of 195 sutras called *The Yoga Sutras.* These sutras create a tapestry of information on everything a yoga practitioner needs to know, how to conduct oneself in society, as well as how to achieve enlightenment. Patanjali, a follower of the Samkhya School, believes in Prakriti and Purusha. In his yoga sutras he presents the Eight Limbed Path of Yoga (see earlier). Patanjali's concepts dominated yoga thought for many centuries (Feuerstein, 2001, pp. 213–254).

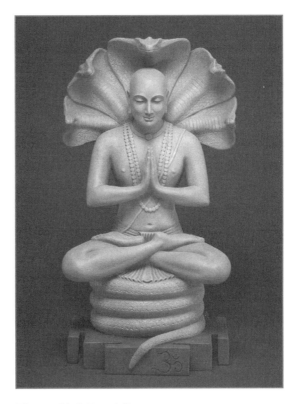

Figure 14-2 Patanjali

1000–1893 A.D.   Post-classical yoga focuses on present reality and teaches one to accept and live in the moment. The belief of the body as a temple is rekindled, and attention to the importance of asana is reestablished. Yoga technique is practiced to transform the body and make it immortal (Feuerstein, 2001, pp. 257–278).

1200–1300 A.D.   The sage Svatmarama compiles a practical treatise on yoga called the *Hathayoga Pradipika*. It gives guidelines to beginners on the journey from the physical body to the spiritual. This classic manual included information about yoga asanas, *pranayama*, and other yoga concepts (Feuerstein, 2001, pp. 30). Many modern schools of Hatha Yoga have been influenced by the *Hathayoga Pradipika*, including Iyengar yoga and Ashtanga yoga.

YOGA IN AMERICA

1893   Modern Western yoga begins at the Parliament of Religion in Chicago. During this meeting, Swami Vivekananda from India introduces Americans to yoga. He tours the United States, giving inspirational lectures. Many yoga masters later cross the ocean and continue to spread yoga all over the United States (Yogananda, 1993, pp. 542–543).

1920   Paramahansa Yogananda (**Figure 14-3**) comes to the United States and lectures about the science of yoga and the teachings of healthy living. He states that by practicing kriya yoga, devotion and service, one can achieve a direct experience of the Divine. Yogananda, known for his book, *The Autobiography of a Yogi*, and his organization, the Self Realization Fellowship, spread his teachings of yoga and meditation (Yogananada, 1993, pp. 399–407).

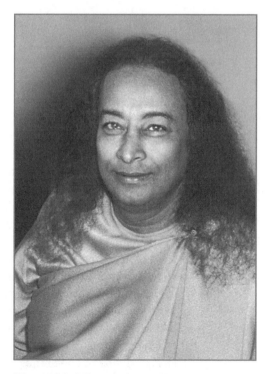

Figure 14-3 Paramahansa Yogananda

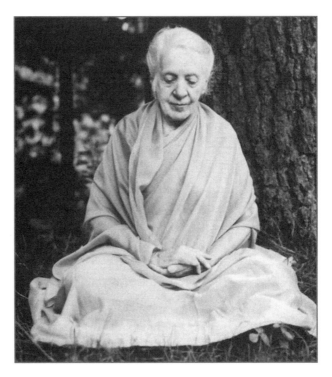

Figure 14-4 Indra Devi

1947	"Hatha" Yoga debuts in Hollywood, California, with the opening of a yoga studio by Russian-born Indra Devi (**Figure 14–4**). She teaches many movie stars and educates hundreds of yoga teachers.
1961	Hatha Yoga appears on American television with Richard Hittleman, and his book, *The Twenty-Eight Day Yoga Plan*, sells millions of copies.
1962	Maharishi Mahesh Yogi teaches the Transcendental Meditation program™ and yoga to The Beatles, giving yoga and meditation a promotional boost. The Transcendental Meditation program™ can only be learned from a qualified, certified instructor in a series of face-to-face small group instructional settings. Meditation can be relaxing (**Figure 14–5**).
1966	B. K. S. Iyengar, one of the premier yogis responsible for introducing yoga to the West, publishes his interna-

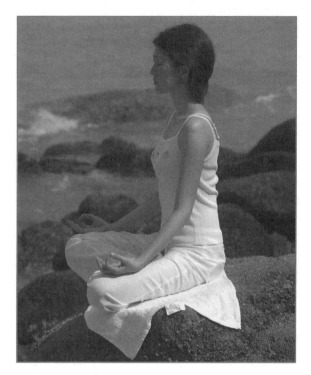

Figure 14-5 Meditation

tional best-selling book, *Light on Yoga*. This book contains photographs and descriptions of many yoga postures. It presents his theories of yoga, known now as Iyengar yoga (Iyengar, 1979, pp. 13–14). B. K. S. Iyengar is 90 years old and still teaches and practices yoga.

2007   Modern yoga teachers continue to expand our knowledge of yoga. A few of these master teachers are Ganga White (**Figure 14-6**), Erich Shiffmann, Shiva Rea, John Friend, and Seane Corn (**Figure 14-7**).

Present   **You** as a yoga student influence and impact your family, community, and the world!

Evolving for thousands of years, yoga is a living system, continuing to grow with each yogi's contributions.

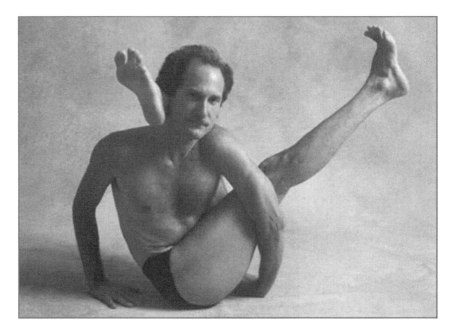

Figure 14-6 Ganga White

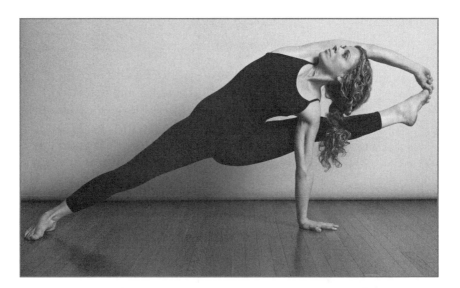

Figure 14-7 Seane Corn

STUDY QUESTIONS

1. What were the initial goals of the yoga postures?
2. Describe each of the five branches of yoga.
3. What is the meaning of:
    a. Yoga?
    b. Asana?
    c. *Pranayama*?
4. What does the term *Hatha Yoga* mean? From which two limbs of the Eight-Limbed Path did Hatha Yoga originate?
5. From the descriptions, which style of Hatha Yoga appeals to you and why?
6. What are two ancient yoga texts and what significance did each have on the development of yoga philosophy?
7. Who is *the father of yoga* and what was his main contribution to yoga?

 # YOGA MOMENT

Observe how you incorporate bhakti, jnana, karma, raja, and Tantra yoga in your own life. Record these observations.

CHAPTER FIFTEEN

Reap the Benefits of Yoga

Radiate Health!

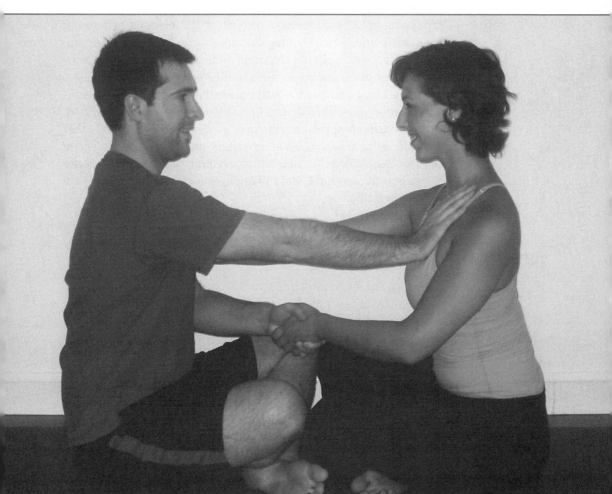

Basketball is an endurance sport, and you have to learn to control your breath; that's the essence of yoga, too. So, I consciously began using yoga techniques in my practice and playing. I think yoga helped reduce the number and severity of injuries I suffered. As preventative medicine, it's unequaled.

— Kareem Abdul-Jabbar

Make yoga a habit. Practice *pranayama* and *asanas* consistently, using correct alignment, strength, and grace. Watch changes occur in your life on a daily basis and long term. By understanding how yoga affects our lives, our appreciation of the mind–body connection is enhanced and the desire to practice yoga daily increases.

Throughout this book we have described the obvious benefits of yoga: stretching and strengthening the body's musculature, sharpening concentration, and quieting the mind. These benefits can easily be experienced after just a few yoga sessions. The benefits are also relative to the postures being practiced. A well-rounded practice includes asanas from each category described (standing, seated, prone, supine, inverted, and restorative). Beyond the benefits previously described, many other transformations occur as a result of consistent practice. *A Physiological Handbook for Teachers of Yogasana* by Mel Robin describes the science behind yoga and the dramatic and subtle physiological and psychological effects of the practice.

PHYSIOLOGICAL BENEFITS

- All the forward, backward, and twisting spinal movements keep the spine healthy. They improve the circulation of nutrients into, and the removal of waste products from, the spinal column, thereby forestalling the premature decalcification of the spine. When the spine remains supple and elongated, the vertebrae do not collapse upon one another and cause pain and nerve damage (Robin, 2002, pp. 82–83).
- Spinal flexion and extension compress and stimulate the internal organs. The pressure that is applied to these organs, specifically the

abdominal organs, aids in digestion and healthy elimination (Lidell, 1983, pp. 182).

- The yoga breath involves the abdominal muscles as well as the diaphragm. This involvement compresses the visceral organs on the inhale and releases the pressure during the exhale. This action massages the internal organs, supports blood flow through the organs, and promotes peristalsis, which is the wave of muscle contractions that transports food and waste through the intestines (Robin, 2002, pp. 371).

- Yoga asanas balance the active aspect of the nervous system, the sympathetic, with the relaxing aspect, the parasympathetic. This creates equilibrium in the nervous system that generates a deep sense of relaxation and lowers stress levels (Robin, 2002, pp. 157–159).

- Stretching performed in yoga promotes the formulation of new capillaries. This increases circulation to the body. This increase in circulation speeds healing and strengthens the areas against injury and disease (Robin, 2002, pp. 177).

- Yoga practice builds a stronger, more dense bone mass. Weight bearing is experienced on all body parts—even the head. The length of time each asana is held is also conducive to building bone mass (Robin, 2002, pp. 241).

- Hypertension, or high blood pressure, heart rate, and respiration decrease with consistent asana practice. The efficiency of the heart increases, helping to prevent coronary heart disease (Robin, 2002, pp. 337).

- Full body inversions improve drainage of body fluids from the legs toward the heart. This reverse flow of fluids aids conditions such as fatigue, migraines, headaches, indigestion, constipation, diabetes, sexual malfunction, varicose veins, hemorrhoids, depression, anxiety, tension, and insomnia (Robin, 2002, pp. 349).

- Yoga has been shown to boost the immune system. First, it promotes the formation of red and white blood cells. It also increases the circulation of body fluids. This regular circulation ensures that all body sites are visited regularly by the mobile components of the immune system. Second, yoga not only speeds the delivery of disease-fighting cells, it also builds high levels of the immune component cells (Robin, 2002, pp. 390).

- Circulation to the thyroid gland increases when performing inversions. This helps to regulate the body's metabolism and also lowers blood cholesterol (Lidell, 1983, pp. 185–186).

- Increased circulation to the pancreas during yoga practice helps stabilize blood sugar levels (Lidell, 1983, pp. 186).
- Increased circulation through asana practice affects male and female reproductive organs, aiding in relieving many disorders (Lidell, 1983, pp. 184–186).

PSYCHOLOGICAL BENEFITS

- Yoga strengthens the endocrine glands, especially the pineal gland, the producer of the hormone, melatonin. This helps to balance both parts of the nervous system, the **sympathetic nervous system**, the fight or flight aspect, with the **parasympathetic nervous system**, the relaxing aspect. This balance improves memory and decreases anxiety (Robin, 2002, pp. 404).
- Back-bending sequences combat depression. These chest-opening asanas stimulate the sympathetic nervous system, bringing energy and vitality to the body. Consequently, mood is elevated (Robin, 2002, pp. 467).
- Forward-bending asanas relax the frontal brain. This quiets the nervous system (Robin, 2002, pp. 215).
- Anxiety and stress levels can be lessened through the practice of yoga. The relaxing asanas promote the parasympathetic response while inhibiting the sympathetic aspect of the nervous system (Robin, 2002, pp. 471). Reducing stress levels has been shown to strengthen the immune system as well as prevent heart disease.

BRINGING YOGA INTO YOUR DAILY LIFE

Like a house protecting one from the heat of the sun, Hatha Yoga protects the practitioner.

— ***Hatha Yoga Pradipika*, ancient yoga text**

Yoga positively impacts personal relationships, work, eating and sleeping habits, and virtually every daily task. Yoga practitioners create a ripple effect by spreading their consciousness, peace, and creativity into the community and the world! Yoga philosophy declares *one centered yogi effects thousands of people.*

Examples of life transformations through yoga are:

*   *Family relationships*: Yoga teaches patience and calmness, important tools for dealing with relationships. Parents report less reactivity and more creativity when dealing with their children. Communications with a spouse or loved one are clearer, more concise, and more honest.
*   *Conscious food choices*: After a yoga practice, charged with positive energy, choosing healthy foods is a natural outcome. A yogi's diet consists of natural and unprocessed foods. Yogis consistently hydrate their bodies because they understand the importance of water for healthy body processes. This awareness of nutrition positively affects the family's eating habits.
*   *Serving humanity*: When consistently practicing yoga, an individual may become more empathetic and desire to help those less fortunate. The attitude of gratitude grows. Volunteering in the community can be a natural outgrowth of the yogi's view of oneness.
*   *Positive thinking*: Science teaches us that our thoughts create our reality. When we practice yoga, we feel better about ourselves. We are more positive about our approach to life. This self-appreciation expresses itself in how we live our lives, how we relate to others, how we accomplish our goals, and how we overcome obstacles.
*   *Developing compassion*: The physical practice of yoga opens the heart, not only the muscle of the heart with its four chambers and vessels, but the heart of love and kindness. It teaches appreciation, which makes one more accepting of others.
*   *Self-love and acceptance*: In a yoga class, every body is unique. We all have different genetics, different bone structure, different emotionality, and different histories. Yoga is noncompetitive, so it encourages self-love and acceptance.
*   *Respect of self and others*: Yoga teaches respect: respect your limitations, respect the other people in the class, and respect the instructor. This attitude infuses into daily life and all the people we encounter.
*   *Role model of radiant health*: The body is energy. As one becomes healthier, the body becomes more vibrant. This radiance affects others.
*   *Feeling more relaxed*: In our fast-paced world, where we move at half the speed of light, learning to relax is an art. Consistent yoga

practice teaches relaxation. It encourages a deeper enjoyment of life and buffers stressful situations.

" Student Testimonial

"Yoga helps me discover an inner calmness and a sense of peace. It also helps me trust my own strength, on and off the mat, and face challenges while being gentle and patient with myself."

Yoga is a journey. Life is a journey. We encounter easy paths on the journey as well as difficult challenges. The tools developed through yoga—strength, balance, poise, grace, calmness, courage, and patience—assist an individual through the journey.

STUDY QUESTIONS

1. What are two physiological changes resulting from regular yoga practice?
2. What are two psychological benefits resulting from regular yoga practice?
3. What are three ways to bring yoga into your daily life?
4. Write your own testimonial on the ways yoga has positively impacted your life.

YOGA MOMENT

Observe yourself in the course of a day. What are three ways that yoga practice has affected your daily life? Record your observations.

Yoga Guidelines for Special Populations

Respect Yourself and Others

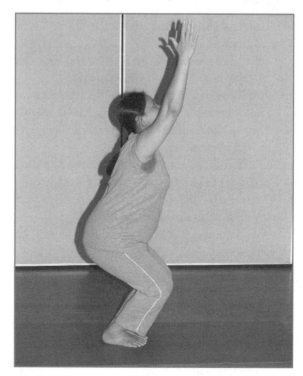

PREGNANCY AND POSTPARTUM

The **holistic** nature of yoga benefits the pregnant and postpartum woman. The asanas stretch, strengthen, and soothe the muscles and joints. Yoga breathing energizes, focuses, and relaxes the body and mind. This combination affects not only the pregnancy but also the labor, delivery, and recovery.

Guidelines Before You Begin Your Yoga Practice

- Check with your doctor for permission to participate in a yoga class. Be aware of any necessary modifications.
- Inform your yoga instructor that you are pregnant and of your due date.
- Read books on yoga and pregnancy so that you know the precautions and modifications to take with poses as you move through your first, second, and third trimesters.

Basic Guidelines

- Keep hydrated throughout the class. Do not allow your body to get overheated.
- Avoid asanas on the back after the first trimester. These poses can restrict blood flow to the uterus.
- Avoid over-stretching. The ligaments are soft and are more susceptible to strains and pulls because of hormonal changes.
- During the second and third trimesters, avoid asanas that put weight on the abdomen.
- During the second and third trimesters, avoid strenuous abdominal poses such as yoga sit-ups and Boat pose.
- During the second and third trimesters, avoid twists because the lower back is more vulnerable.
- Avoid shoulder stands, headstands, and handstands. These invert the uterus.
- Rest on your left side for Savasana with a blanket under your knees and another under the head.
- Do not hold the breath for a long time. This restricts oxygen to the fetus.

Practicing yoga not only affects the overall physical vitality, mental awareness, and peace of mind of the pregnant woman, it also affects the health of the developing fetus and the recovering mother.

Beneficial Aspects of the Yoga Practice

- Breathing and *pranayama*: This brings life-sustaining oxygen to mother and baby and helps with overall physical and emotional fitness. Proper breathing can be a vital tool during labor and delivery!
- Yoga asanas: These positions gently stretch and strengthen the entire body, especially the area of the pelvic floor and abdominal muscles, preparing the woman for labor and childbirth. The asanas support good circulation and the flow of nutrients to both the mom and the growing baby. The yoga asanas also teach and maintain correct alignment. This is helpful as the woman's body gains weight and the fetus grows.
- Meditation: This quietude establishes mindfulness and reduces anxiety and worry often associated with the changes that occur during pregnancy and recovery.
- Restorative poses: These rejuvenating asanas bring the mind, body, and spirit into harmony. This allows deep rest and relaxation to the nervous system and creates an openness of heart and an expansion of consciousness.
- Practicing yoga in a prenatal yoga class: This builds a support system with other pregnant women and women with new babies.

Suggested Readings

Yoga for Pregnancy, Birth, and Beyond, by Francoise Freedman and Doriel Hall
Pregnancy Perfection, by Pamela L. Dusymski
Step by Step Yoga for Pregnancy: Essentials, by Wendy Teasedill
Preparing for Birth with Yoga, by Janet Balaskas

DVDs for Your Home Yoga Practice

"Yoga for Pregnancy" by *Yoga Journal*
"Prenatal Yoga with Shiva Rea"

OVERWEIGHT PERSONS

Congratulations for finding yoga! This scientific tool of exercise can help you transform your body and your life. Weight gain occurs when the food intake exceeds the energy output. These extra calories that are eaten but not burned are turned into fat. Obesity strains the respiratory system, the circulatory system, the digestive system, and the nervous system. Weight loss, increased energy, and more vitality are outcomes of practicing yoga, proper breathing, and meditation.

Guidelines for Yoga Practice If Overweight

- Obtain permission from your doctor. Find out if there are any poses you should not perform.
- Tell your yoga instructor about any conditions you have, including eye conditions. Also inform the instructor of any medications you take.
- Go slowly. Move with awareness, breath, and consciousness.
- Practice yoga at least three times a week. Your body benefits from even a short practice at home.
- Practice yoga properly under the guidance of a certified instructor. Utilize appropriate modifications.

Yoga Works in Many Ways

- Reducing stress: The postures work on the nervous system to rejuvenate the body's energy systems and to calm and clear the mind.
- Increasing the metabolic rate: Yoga asana practice can increase your caloric need to burn fat stores in the body. Practice modified Sun Salutations to create heat in the body and burn calories. Minimize or eliminate television watching and other sedentary activities. Practice yoga instead!
- Change in lifestyle: The yoga philosophy of nonviolence carries over directly to oneself—no harm to the body temple. Yogis choose healthy food and drinks and a lifestyle that supports health and well-being.
- Awareness: Practicing meditation (see Chapter 3) every day can boost spirits and create a sense of calm. As you discover inner stillness, emotional stability grows and emotional eating lessens.

- Community: Compulsive overeating and frequent snacking sometimes occur due to stress, loneliness, and boredom. Spend time with other yoga students for support and encouragement. The friends you make in yoga class positively influence your life.
- Relaxation: Meditation, mindfulness, restorative yoga poses, and deep relaxation (see Chapter 12) create peace and well-being from the inside out. Incorporate these into your daily life.

Suggested Readings

Yoga, A Path to Holistic Health, by B. K. S. Iyengar
Peaceful Weight Loss Through Yoga, by Brandt Bhanu Passalaccqua

OLDER ADULTS

The older adult can prevent and alleviate many of the health challenges of aging by practicing yoga. Senior yoga classes in private studios and colleges continue to grow in popularity. The union of mind, body, and spirit, along with the health benefits of yoga, makes this a popular form of movement for the senior citizen.

Guidelines to Follow for the Active Older Adult

- Know your limitations and inform your instructor of your limitations.
- Be constantly aware of correct alignment.
- Move gently and slowly in the transitions between poses.
- If you have osteoporosis, avoid poses that require forward spinal flexion, twists, and lateral flexion.
- Reduce the time that each asana is held.
- Practice asanas that encourage spinal stabilization.
- Practice yoga mudras (hand positions) at every practice provide fine motor conditioning for the hands.
- Rest whenever you feel fatigued or unsteady.
- Use a chair or a wall for balance poses.
- Focus on asanas specifically for the ankles, hips, hamstrings, low back, and chest muscles because these areas are typically weak in the older adult.

- Practice *pranayama* and meditation regularly, along with the asanas.

    Scientific studies describe the positive impact of yoga on the geriatric population. Some of these findings include:

- Improved sleep patterns
- Improved hand strength in arthritic patients
- Better blood sugar control and improved lung capacity in diabetics
- Decrease in blood pressure and cholesterol levels
- Reduction in weight gain
- Improved mood and lessened anxiety
- Decrease in chronic pain
- Decrease in breathing difficulties

The old saying goes, "if you don't use it, you lose it!" Yoga keeps you young!!

Suggested Readings

The New Yoga for People Over 50: A Comprehensive Guide for Midlife and Older Beginners, by Suza Francina
Yoga for the Young at Heart, by Susan Winter Ward

Nutrition to Complement the Yoga Lifestyle

Feed Your Soul

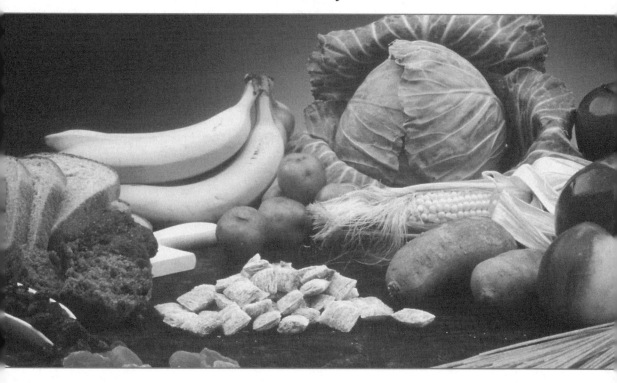

A healthy lifestyle is composed of exercising, constructively relieving stress, having passion in your life, committing to relationships, and eating well. What does eating to maintain a healthy lifestyle mean? Outlined below are ways to keep your eating habits healthy:

- Choose natural foods, preferably organically grown. Avoid processed foods.
- Avoid foods containing artificial colorings and preservatives.
- Choose locally grown vegetables and fruits.
- Eat a variety of foods.
- Avoid sodas and drink lots of water.
- Make sure your diet contains all of the six important nutrients.

SIX IMPORTANT NUTRIENTS

Protein builds and repairs muscle tissue. It is required to make hemoglobin, which carries oxygen to the cells. Our diet should consist of 12% to 20% protein. One gram of protein equals four calories. Protein is made up of building blocks called **amino acids**. Of the 22 amino acids in protein, eight are essential. These essential amino acids cannot be manufactured in the body and therefore must be supplied by the food we eat. There are two types of protein: animal protein (all meat, fish, chicken, eggs, milk, and milk products) and plant protein (legumes, tofu, nuts, and grains). Animal protein contains all the essential amino acids, making it a complete protein. Plant proteins do not contain all the essential amino acids, so they must be appropriately combined to be complete. Examples of combining plant proteins are beans and corn, rice and beans; beans and noodles; and black-eyed peas and rice.

Carbohydrates are used solely for energy production. Our diet should consist of between 50% and 60% carbohydrates. One gram of carbohydrate equals four calories. Although all carbohydrates have certain chemistry in common, there is a difference between one carbohydrate and another. Simple carbohydrates—sugar—are ingested and converted to blood glucose immediately. This can cause blood glucose levels to fluctuate rapidly, making energy levels vacillate. These sweet carbohydrates offer no nutritional value. Complex carbohydrates are the natural sugars found in fruits, vegetables, bread, pasta, cereal, potatoes, and rice. They are the best source of energy because they convert blood glucose slowly and supply a sustained energy output. Complex carbohydrates contain high levels of vitamins, minerals, and fiber.

Fat supplies energy and fuel to the body both at rest and during exercise. It also provides cushioning for the body's vital organs and protection from extreme cold temperatures. Our diet should consist of 20% to 30% fat. Dietary fats have the highest energy content of all nutrients, at nine calories per gram! There are two types of fat. The healthy type is called "unsaturated" and is liquid at room temperature. It includes all vegetable oils, nuts, and avocados. The unhealthy type of fat is called "saturated" and is hard at room temperature. This includes all animal fat and animal products such as eggs, dairy items, butter, lard, margarine, palm oil, and cottonseed oil. This type of fat should be avoided because it clogs arteries and increases cholesterol.

Vitamins assist the body to use and absorb proteins, carbohydrates, and fats. Vitamins are essential for the body's normal metabolic functioning. Choose a rainbow variety of fruits and vegetables to ensure that your diet is rich in vitamins. There are two types of vitamins. Water-soluble vitamins include all the B vitamins and vitamin C. These are excreted in the urine and therefore are not stored in appreciable amounts. It is important to replenish these vitamins daily. Fat-soluble vitamins include A, D, E, and K. They tend to remain stored in the body and are usually not excreted through the urine. An excess of these vitamins can be toxic to the body.

Minerals are the building materials for body tissues and serve as nerve regulators. Like vitamins, they help use and absorb the other nutrients. Iron and calcium are two minerals especially important for women. Iron is found in hemoglobin, which is a protein molecule that carries blood to the muscles. A lack of iron in the diet can induce anemia, especially during the menstrual cycle when blood is lost. Calcium is necessary for muscle contraction. A lack of calcium means the body will take the calcium from the bones to contract the muscles. Eventually, this process can lead to osteoporosis, a bone-weakening disease. All minerals except iron are excreted by the body after they have carried out their function. Therefore, minerals must be replenished daily.

Water is second to oxygen in sustaining life. It is necessary for all energy production in the body, for temperature control, and for the elimination of waste products. Water makes up 80% of our body. A person can live for weeks without food, but it is a miracle if they can live without water for a week. It is recommended to drink at least half of one's body weight in ounces of water per day. This means that a 120-pound person should drink at least 60 ounces of water a day. Use glass or safe plastics—avoiding Bisphenol-A (BPA) plastics—to hold your water.

A diet that does not include all these nutrients can have long-term negative effects (Fallon, 2001). Use Worksheet 5, Nutrition Diary, to record your daily diet. Determine whether all these nutrients are included. Make intelligent changes to your diet if it does not contain these six important nutrients.

SUGGESTED READING

Prescription for Nutritional Healing, by Phyllis A. Balch and James F. Balch, MD
Nancy Clark's Sports Nutrition Guidebook, by Nancy Clark
Yogic Nutrition, by Dr. Gin L. Nick
Healing with Whole Foods, by Paul Pitchford

Yoga Resources

Acknowledge Your Achievements

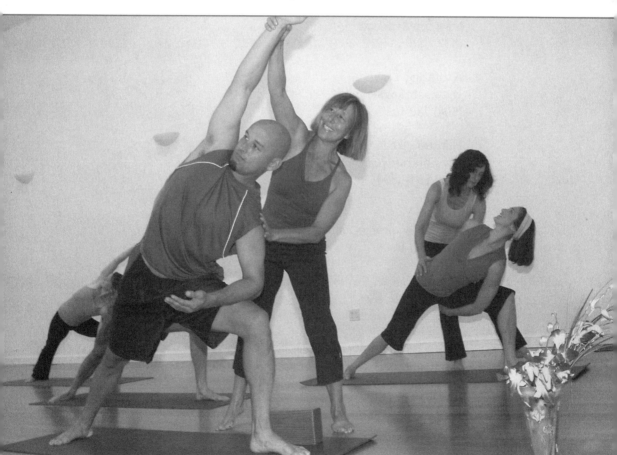

AUTHOR CONTACTS

Minda Goodman Kraines
MindaGKraines@aol.com
Visit www.missioncollege.org for class schedules.

Barbara Rose Sherman
Visit www.barbararosesherman.com for information on workshops,
retreats, and classes.

CERTIFIED YOGA SCHOOLS AND TEACHER TRAININGS
Anusara
www.anusara.com
(888) 398-9642

Ashtanga Yoga
www.ashtanga.com
(604) 732-6111

Bikram's Yoga College of India
www.bikramyoga.com
(310) 854-5800

Iyengar Yoga
www.iyengar-yoga.com
(415) 753-0909

Kripalu Center for Yoga and Health
www.kripalu.org
(800) 741-7353

Santa Barbara Yoga Center
www.santabarbarayogacenter.com
(805) 965-6045

International Sivananda Yoga Vedanta Centres
www.sivananda.org
(800) 783-9642

White Lotus Foundation
www.whitelotus.org
(805) 964-1944

Yoga Alliance
www.yogaalliance.org
(877) 964-2255

Yoga Works
www.yogaworks.com
(310) 664-6470

MINDA'S FAVORITE YOGA CDS

"Yoga on Sacred Ground," by Chinmaya Dunster
"Union," by Rasa
"Hotel Tara 2—The Intimate Side of Buddha-Lounge," by Sequoia
Grove

BARBARA'S FAVORITE YOGA CDS

"Love Is Space," by Deva Premal
"Music for Yoga," by Steven Halpren
"Reiki Whale Song," by Kamal

Suggested Reading

Discover Yes and Zest Moments

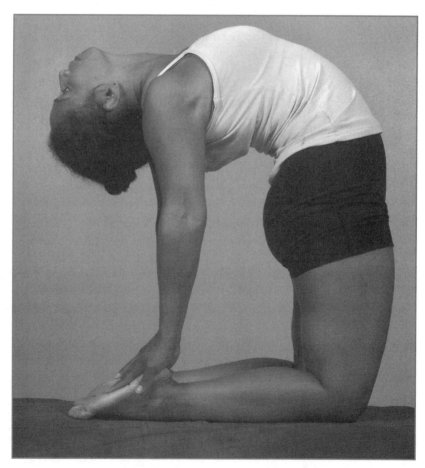

There are a myriad of books written about yoga philosophy, asanas, and breathing. We have just included our favorites. All the books we have listed are inspiring, well-written, and informative. Enjoy!

Anatomy of Hatha Yoga: A Manual for Students, Teachers and Practitioners, by H. David Coulter
This book goes into beautiful detail on all the musculature and physiological aspects of the asanas. It is very scientific, but well worth a read.

Autobiography of a Yogi, by Paramahansa Yogananda
This book is the epic tale of Yogananda's life and teachings.

Light on Yoga: The Bible of Modern Yoga, by B. K. S. Iyengar and Yehudi Menuhin
Iyengar is the premier yogi master. This truly is the yoga bible, discussing every aspect of the yoga practice.

Meditations from the Mat: Daily Reflections on the Path of Yoga, by Rolf Gate and Katrina Kenison
This includes 365 philosophical quotes and introspective passages to begin your day or yoga practice.

Peace Is in Every Step, by Tich Nhat Hahn
This book inspires mindfulness in daily life.

Relax and Renew, by Judith Lassester
This book describes in detail a variety of restorative yoga poses.

The Little Book of Yoga Breathing: Pranayama Made Easy, by Scott Shaw
This is a great, small book on yoga breathing techniques.

Yoga: The Path to Holistic Health, by B. K. S. Iyengar
While expensive and large, the photographs are fabulous and make this book a must-read.

Yoga the Iyengar Way, by Silva, Mira, and Shyam Mehta
This book includes beautiful photographs and clear descriptions of yoga asanas.

Yoga as Medicine, by *Yoga Journal* and Timothy McCall
This text dives deeply into the science of yoga and all the health issues it can benefit.

Yoga: The Spirit and Practice of Moving Into Stillness, by Erich Schiffmann
Erich's inspiring book encourages mindful meditation and asana practice to allow students to experience the heart of yoga.

Yoga Beyond Belief, by Ganga White
Yoga master Ganga White goes beyond the asanas to share his insights and philosophy of yoga.

Medical Profile

Name _____ Date _____

Age _____ Day/Time Class Meets _____

Local Address _____

Home Phone _____ Cell Phone _____

Have you had previous instruction in yoga? _____

       If yes, how long and where? _____

Are you currently involved in a regular exercise program? _____

       If yes, what type of activity? _____

Please list the reasons you are taking this course:

Please identify personal goals you wish to achieve in this course:

Please check the appropriate space if you have the condition listed. Add comments if the condition would limit your participation in the yoga practice:

____ allergies   ____ dysmenorrhea   ____ high blood pressure

____ arthritis   ____ epilepsy   ____ muscular injuries

____ asthma   ____ eye problems   ____ pregnancy

____ diabetes   ____ heart disease   ____ other (please explain)

Do you take any medication on a regular basis? _____

If so, indicate what type and if it will affect your practice. _____

Emergency Contact Name and Phone Number _____

I am aware of my medical profile and will proceed safely in my yoga practice.

Signature _____ Date _____

Evaluating and Monitoring Your Flexibility

Name _____ Class Day/Time _____

Perform these exercises with a partner if possible to evaluate your flexibility at the beginning of the class term. Repeat the same exercises at the end of the term. You will need two soft tape measures to complete the evaluations. Be aware that flexibility is specific to each joint in the body and even to each side of the body for the same joint. With consistent yoga practice you will see an improvement in your flexibility.

EVALUATION FOR HAMSTRINGS AND LOWER BACK

- Using masking tape, secure two soft tape measures on the floor. Start at a wall and place them parallel about 30 inches apart (far enough apart so you can sit in between them).

- Remove your shoes and socks. Sit between the tape measures with the soles of the feet flat against a wall.

- Sitting erect, place the fingertips next to your hips.

- Slide the hands down the tape measures and record how many inches your fingertips are from the wall. Keep the knees fully extended and the soles of the feet flat against the wall.

- If you can touch the wall, record that information.

_____ Initial Assessment _____ Final Assessment

EVALUATION FOR HIP JOINT AND INNER THIGHS

- Place one tape measure on the floor, extending out from the wall.

- Sit in the middle of the tape measure with the legs spread as wide as possible and the inner edges of the feet against the wall.

- Measure the distance your groin is from the wall.

_____ Initial Assessment _____ Final Assessment

EVALUATION FOR QUADRICEPS AND HIP FLEXORS

• Lie on the stomach.

• Stretch the left arm forward on the floor with the palm down and place the forehead on the floor.

• Grab the right foot with the right hand and pull the heel toward the buttocks.

• Measure the distance between the heel and the buttocks.

• Repeat with the left leg.

_____ Initial Assessment Right   _____ Final Assessment Right

_____ Initial Assessment Left   _____ Final Assessment Left

EVALUATION FOR THE SHOULDER JOINT

• Stand in good alignment with the feet in a comfortable stance.

• Bring the left arm up and pat the back. The left elbow will point upward.

• With the right arm down and the palm facing the back, bend the right elbow and slide the hand across the back to reach for the left fingers.

• Using the tape measure, measure the distance between the two hands. If the fingers clasp or even touch, make that observation.

• Repeat on the other side.

_____ Initial Assessment Right   _____ Final Assessment Right

_____ Initial Assessment Left   _____ Final Assessment Left

Evaluating Your Posture

Correct posture creates the foundation for Tadasana as described in Chapter 4. This alignment is appropriate for standing, walking, running, and even sitting. Use the guidelines in the evaluations below to help you analyze your current natural posture. Reevaluate your natural posture at the end of your yoga course or eight to ten weeks into your yoga practice.

A wall mirror will be needed for this evaluation. If a partner is available, he or she can help with the evaluation.

In yoga clothing and barefoot, stand in your natural posture in front of the mirror.

1. Face sideways and check the following details: draw an imaginary line at the middle of the ear, at the middle of the shoulder, at the center of the hip, just behind the kneecap, and in front of the ankle. The line should be straight and vertical.

    Where does your posture deviate from the straight line?

    _____ Initial Evaluation

    _____ Final Evaluation

2. Observe the natural curves of the spine. There should be a mild inward curve at the cervical spine (behind the neck) and the lumbar spine (lower back). The thoracic spine should be slightly curved outward (see Figure 4-7 in Chapter 4).

    Where does your spine deviate from these curvatures?

    _____ Initial Evaluation

    _____ Final Evaluation

3. Face forward and check the following details: Your shoulders, hips, and knees should be on the same plane. A horizontal line should be able to be drawn from one side to the other.

    Where does your posture deviate from these points?

    _____ Initial Evaluation

    _____ Final Evaluation

4. Face forward and check if the kneecaps face forward.

   What direction do your kneecaps face?

   _____ Initial Evaluation   _____ Final Evaluation

5. The ankles should be directly above the feet, not rolling inward or outward.

   What position do your ankles follow?

   _____ Initial Evaluation   _____ Final Evaluation

6. Face forward and check that your head is balanced with the ears equal distance from the shoulders.

   What deviations do you observe?

   _____ Initial Evaluation   _____ Final Evaluation

After you have completed all six steps in the initial and final evaluations, summarize the results. Be attentive to any areas that need work by practicing Tadasana on a regular basis.

Personal Yoga Practice Log

Make copies of this page so you can record home practices throughout the course.

Name _____ Date _____ Duration of Practice _____

Asanas Practiced _____

_____

_____

_____

Observations About Practice _____

_____

_____

_____

Name _____ Date _____ Duration of Practice _____

Asanas Practiced _____

_____

_____

_____

Observations About Practice _____

_____

_____

_____

Nutrition Diary

Become aware of your daily diet by keeping a nutrition diary. This allows you to observe your eating habits and to create change where appropriate. To get the most out of this diary, record your food intake after each meal for a whole week. Make copies of the chart provided and fill it in completely for one week.

FOLLOW THESE TIPS

- Do not change your eating habits while using this diary.
- Tell the truth.
- Write down *everything*.
- Be specific.

HOW TO FILL IN THE CHART

- How much: Indicate the amount of food eaten. Estimate the volume (½ cup), the weight (2 ounces), and/or the number of food items consumed.
- What kind: Write down the type of food. Be specific. Include sauces and gravies. Write down the extras, such as soda, salad dressing, and mayonnaise.
- Time: Write down the time you ate.
- Where: Write down where you ate, what room in your house, what restaurant, or in the car.
- Who: Write down if you ate alone or with whom.
- Mood: How did you feel while you were eating, happy, sad, depressed, etc.?

Here is an example of how to fill out the diary.

Food and Drink					
How Much	**What Kind**	**Time**	**Where**	**With Whom**	**Mood**
3	Oatmeal cookies	3 P.M.	Office	Alone	Bored
4 oz.	Tuna fish	6 P.M.	Kitchen	Mom	Tired
2 slices	Whole wheat bread	6 P.M.	Kitchen	Mom	Tired
1 TBS	Mayonnaise	6 P.M.	Kitchen	Mom	Tired
1 cup	Green peas	6 P.M.	Kitchen	Mom	Tired
3 oz.	Chocolate	11 P.M.	Study	Alone	Worried

Date:					
Food and Drink					
How Much	**What Kind**	**Time**	**Where**	**With Whom**	**Mood**

Glossary

Amino acids   building blocks of protein. There are 22 essential amino acids that make up a complete protein.

Arthritis   a medical condition affecting a joint or joints, causing pain, swelling, and stiffness.

Asanas   postures used in yoga.

Bhakti   derived from the Sanskrit word *bhaj*, which means "to serve." Bhakti yoga is the yoga of devotion and selfless love.

Drishti   the focus point that is necessary during the practice of yoga asanas.

Endorphins   hormones found in the brain that create an elated feeling and a sense of well-being. These hormones are produced during yoga.

Glaucoma   an eye disorder marked by abnormally high pressure within the eyeball that leads to damage of the optic disc and, if not treated, causes impaired vision and sometimes blindness.

Hatha   *Ha* means "sun" and *tha* means "moon." It is also the union of opposites and the physical aspect of yoga.

Holistic   including or involving all of something—especially all of someone's physical, mental, and social conditions, not just physical symptoms—in the treatment of illness.

Hypertension   abnormally high blood pressure.

Jhana   in Sanskrit the word *jhana* means "knowledge" or "wisdom." Jhana yogis study the scriptures and texts to reach enlightenment.

Karma   the Hindu and Buddhist philosophy according to which the quality of people's current and future lives is determined by their behavior in this and in previous lives. Karma yoga is living a life of service.

Kyphosis   an excessive curve of the thoracic spine. It gives the appearance of a "hunchback."

Lines of energy   energetic currents that flow through each yoga asana. This helps the body align itself from the inside out.

Lordosis   an excessive inward curving of the spine in the lower part of the back.

Mantra   a sacred word, chant, or sound that is repeated during meditation to facilitate spiritual power and transformation of consciousness.

Nadi shodhana   alternate nostril breathing. *Nadi* is a tubular organ for the passage of energy or *prana*. *Shodhana* means to *purify* or *to cleanse*. Therefore, the *nadi shodhana pranayama* is the *purification of the nerves*.

OM   a sacred syllable that is chanted in Hindu and Buddhist prayers and mantras.

Parasympathetic nervous system   the part of the nervous system that controls involuntary and unconscious bodily functions.

Prakriti   in Sanskrit, *prakriti* is "matter."

Pranayama   techniques of breath control used in the practice of yoga. *Prana* means *life force* and *yama* means *to control*.

Prone   lying on the abdomen with the face downward.

Purusha   in Sanskrit, *purusha* is the "soul" or "self."

Raja   in Sanskrit, *raja* means "royal" and refers to the journey of personal enlightenment through meditation.

Relaxation response   physiological response of the human body to meditation.

Sanskrit   the extinct Indo-European language of ancient India.

Scoliosis   an excessive sideways curve of the spine. It can be structural, which requires surgery to repair, or functional, due to poor postural habits.

Supine   lying on the back with the face upward. The palm of the hand is facing upward or away from the body.

Sympathetic nervous system   the part of the autonomic nervous system that is active during stress or danger and is involved in regulating pulse and blood pressure, dilating pupils, and changing muscle tone.

Tantra   in Sanskrit, *tantra* means "to weave" and denotes continuity. Tantra yogis believe that one's true essence exists in every particle of the universe. They aspire to feel unconditional love, bliss, tenderness, and acceptance for all.

Third eye   an energetic point between the eyebrows associated with expanding consciousness.

Ujjayi   literally, means *victory breath* or *victorious breath*. It is a technique in breathing where the lungs fully expand and the chest puffs outward.

References

American Council on Exercise. (2005 September/October). *Fitness Matters* [newsletter]. Study by Dawn Boehde and John Porcari of the University of Wisconsin at LaCrosse.

Benson, Herbert. (1975). *The Relaxation Response*. New York: Avon Books.

Cullen, Lisa Takeuchi. (2006 January 10). "How to Get Smarter, One Breath at a Time." *Time Magazine.*

Edwards, Scott and Tamson S. McMahon. (2006 Fall). "Growing the Brain through Meditation." *The Harvard Mahoney Neuroscience Institute Letter.*

Fallon, Sally. (2001). *Nourishing Traditions*. Washington, DC: New Trends Publishing.

Feuerstein, Georg. (2001). *The Yoga Tradition*. Prescott, AZ: Hohm Press.

Isaacs, Nora. (2006 June). "Tantra Rising." *Yoga Journal.*

Iyengar, B. K. S. (1979). *Light on Yoga*. New York: Schocken Books.

Kappmeier, Kathy Lee and Diane M. Ambrosini. (2006). *Instructing Hatha Yoga*. Champaign, IL: Human Kinetics.

Kornfield, Jack. (2004). *Meditation for Beginners*. Boulder, CO: Sounds True, Inc.

Kramer, Joel. (1980 May/June). "Yoga as Self-Transformation." *Yoga Journal.*

Kraines, Minda Goodman and Esther Pryor. (2004). *Jump Into Jazz*, Fifth Edition. New York: McGraw-Hill.

Krucoff, Carol. (2000 July 10). "Stress and the Art of Breathing." *Los Angeles Times.*

Lidell, Lucy. (1983). *The Sivananda Companion to Yoga*. London: Gaia Books.

Lipson, Elaine. (1991–2002 Winter). "Yoga Works." *Yoga Journal.*

Marano, Hara Estroff. (2001 July/August). "Depression Doing the Thinking." *Psychology Today Magazine.*

Pryor, Esther and Minda Goodman Kraines. (2000). *Keep Moving! Fitness through Aerobics and Step.* Mountainview, CA: Mayfield Publishing.

Raub, James A. (2002 December). "Psychophysiological Effects of Hatha Yoga on Musculoskeletal and Cardiopulmonary Function: A Literature Review." *The Journal of Alternative and Complementary Medicine.*

Robin, Mel. (2002). *A Physiological Handbook for Teachers of Yogasana.* Tucson, AZ: Fenestra Books.

Schatz, Mary Pullig. (1992). *Back Care Basics.* Berkeley, CA: Rodmell Press.

Schiffmann, Erich. (1996). *Yoga, The Spirit and Practice of Moving Into Stillness.* New York: Pocket Books.

Stein, Joel. (2003 August 4). "Just Say Om." *Time Magazine.*

Vad, Vijay. (2004). *Back RX.* New York: Gotham Books.

Weil, Andrew. (1995). *Spontaneous Healing.* New York: Alfred A. Knopf.

White, Ganga. (2007). *Yoga Beyond Belief.* Berkeley, CA: North Atlantic Books.

Yogananda, Paramahansa. (1993). *The Autobiography of a Yogi, Self Realization Fellowship.* Los Angeles: Crystal Clarity Publishers.

Index

Photo Credits

Chapter 1
Page 1 Courtesy of Shiva Rea. Photo by Dusty Edwards; **page 2** © LiquidLibrary; **page 5** © Anyka/ShutterStock, Inc.; **page 6** © ilker canikligil/ShutterStock, Inc; **page 7 (top left)** © AbleStock; **page 7 (top right)** © Tom Grundy/ShutterStock, Inc.; **page 7 (bottom)** © Joseph Shelton/Dreamstime.com; **page 8** © Janetto/Dreamstime.com; **page 9** © Anson Hung/Shutter-Stock, Inc.

Chapter 2
Page 20 © AbleStock; **page 22, 23** Courtesy of Barbara Rose Sherman; **page 24 (right)** © Ksoloits/Dreamstime.com; **page 24 (left)** © Johanna Goodyear/ShutterStock, Inc.; **page 26, 27** Courtesy of Barbara Rose Sherman

Chapter 3
Page 30 Courtesy of Robert Sturman, Sturman Photography, www.RobertSturmanStudio.com; **page 32** Courtesy of Barbara Rose Sherman

Chapter 4
Page 40 © AbleStock; **page 43** Courtesy of Barbara Rose Sherman

Chapter 6
Page 61 Courtesy of John Friend. Photo by Kelly Haas

Chapter 8
Page 103 Courtesy of Wayne Williams, www.WayneWilliamsStudio.com, from *Yoga Beyond Belief: Insights to Awaken and Deepen Your Practice* by Ganga White, published by North Atlantic Books, © 2007 Ganga White. Reprinted by permission of publisher, www.whitelotus.org

Chapter 9
Page 117 Courtesy of Tracey Rich. Photo by Wayne Williams, www.WayneWilliamsStudio.com

Chapter 11
Page 161 Courtesy of Seane Corn. Photo by Erik Asla

Chapter 13
Page 177 Courtesy of Barbara Rose Sherman

Chapter 14
Page 197 Courtesy of Erich Schiffmann; **page 205** © Andrey Pils/ShutterStock, Inc.; **page 206** Courtesy of Natalia Rosenfeld Art Studio, www.nataliasculpture.com; **page 207** Courtesy of Self-Realization Fellowship, Los Angeles, CA; **page 208** Courtesy of the INDRA DEVI FOUNDATION; **page 209** © Kim Pin Tan/ShutterStock, Inc.; **page 210 (top)** Courtesy of White Lotus Foundation. Photographed by Jake Jacobson; **page 210 (bottom)** Courtesy of Seane Corn

Chapter 15
Page 213 Courtesy of Barbara Rose Sherman

Appendix B
Page 225 Courtesy of National Cancer Institute

Appendix D
Page 233 © Alfred Wekelo/ShutterStock, Inc.

Unless otherwise indicated, all photographs and illustrations are under copyright of Jones and Bartlett Publishers, LLC or were photographed by George Welik.